ALTERNATIVE MEDICINE?

A HISTORY

ROBERTA BIVINS

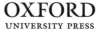

OXFORD
UNIVERSITY PRESS

OXFORD
UNIVERSITY PRESS

Great Clarendon Street, Oxford OX2 6DP

Oxford University Press is a department of the University of Oxford.
It furthers the University's objective of excellence in research, scholarship,
and education by publishing worldwide in

Oxford New York

Auckland Cape Town Dar es Salaam Hong Kong Karachi
Kuala Lumpur Madrid Melbourne Mexico City Nairobi
New Delhi Shanghai Taipei Toronto

With offices in

Argentina Austria Brazil Chile Czech Republic France Greece
Guatemala Hungary Italy Japan Poland Portugal Singapore
South Korea Switzerland Thailand Turkey Ukraine Vietnam

Oxford is a registered trade mark of Oxford University Press
in the UK and in certain other countries

Published in the United States
by Oxford University Press Inc., New York

British Library Cataloguing in Publication Data

Data available

Library of Congress Cataloging in Publication Data

Data available

Typeset by SPI Publisher Services, Pondicherry, India
Printed in Great Britain
on acid-free paper by
Clays Ltd, St. Ives plc

ISBN 978–0–19–921887–5 (Hbk.)
ISBN 978–0–19–954376–2 (Pbk.)

1 3 5 7 9 10 8 6 4 2
2 4 6 8 10 9 7 5 3 1

ALTERNATIVE MEDICINE?

Roberta Bivins is Associate Professor in the Department of History at the University of Warwick. Her work focuses on the transmission of medical expertise between cultures, as exemplified by the transmission of acupuncture to the west, and by the medical experiences of non-western immigrants in multicultural Britain and America.

Praise for *Alternative* Medicine

'A brilliant foil to the privileging of Western medicine...this is cross-cultural history at its best—lively, acute, richly informative, and wonderfully revealing.'
Roger Cooter, Wellcome Trust Centre for the History of Medicine at UCL

'I recommend this book to anyone with more than a passing interest in "alternative" medicine.'
Edzard Ernst, author of *The Desktop Guide to Complementary and Alternative Medicine*

'Ground breaking...Roberta Bivins demonstrates the complex routes that medical knowledge and practice travelled, east to west, north to south, and back again...and disrupts our contemporary notions of "alternative" medicine.'
Allan M. Brandt, author of *The Cigarette Century: The Rise, Fall, and Deadly persistence of the Product that Defined America*

'Well written, concise, yet wide-ranging.'
British Journal for the History of Science

'This well-written and painstakingly researched book would enhance any history of medicine collection.'
Doody's Notes

'[an] elegant and engaging book...Bivins takes us on a fascinating journey from east to west and back again.'
Financial Times

'This compact, densely written history effectively demonstrates how alternative medicine has survived and prospered in the 21st century.'
The Independent

With thanks to the many students whose comments, questions, and complaints have made this a better book

After all, is it necessary to be ever talking of rival systems of medicine, as though scientific truths can possibly vary with the orient of this, that or the other geographical unit? If the one pointed search after truth is everywhere the aim of all scientific endeavour, there can be but one system—one without a second—of any science, whether it be physics, chemistry, biology, medicine or any other. Theories and hypotheses have been and can be many, but truth is one; it is neither eastern or western but universal . . . no true scientist—eastern or western—would ever reject a proposition merely because it was advanced by one born in an orient different from his own . . .

(Muhammad Usman, 1923)

He added that if snakes' blood and crocodiles' teeth produced cures, he would use them.

('Report of the BMA Annual Clinical Meeting', 1968)

PREFACE

I grew up in a world with no 'alternative medicine'. This is not a factor of my age, my culture, or of a particularly conventional upbringing; in fact, rather the reverse. As a child, I shuttled with my academic parents between richly diverse—if somewhat shabby—working-class neighbourhoods in urban New England, a remote village in the far northern Sokoto Caliphate of Nigeria, and the remarkable cities of Kano and Kaduna, also in Nigeria's Muslim north. Whether from a shingle-boarded apartment in the shadow of decaying tower blocks, or from an elegantly domed (but nonetheless mud-built) compound shaded by a mahogany tree, I went out into a world in which 'medicine' took many forms. And although I don't remember my childhood as an unhealthy one, my medical records demonstrate that I was an annoyingly sickly child. Massachusetts winters saw me dangling my feet in municipal emergency rooms, wheezing with pneumonia or silenced by throat infections. In the Nigerian rainy season, I collected parasites and malarias with gay abandon; in the dry season, I replaced them with an exciting range of rashes, infected insect bites, and mysterious fevers.

My Petri dish tendencies were certainly a burden for my mother, but for me they have proven a real boon. I was exposed in childhood to an array of medical practices—no medical system looked particularly strange or 'alternative' to me, because I had no established expectations or assumptions about what was 'normal'. My doctor *du jour* might very well take my temperature, put a stethoscope to my chest, and stick me with needles. On the other hand, I might be carefully catechized about my behaviour just before my illness, have my eyeballs scrutinized, and be given a Koranic amulet to wear against evil spirits. From a child's perspective, the end result was the same: I went home, lay in bed feeling sick for a while, and then felt better. And at least the amulets didn't hurt.

Two medical encounters stand out for me now as particularly influential, and particularly relevant to my understanding of medicine and culture today. The first is an episode in that tiny Nigerian village. I became deathly ill—so sick that a group of nomadic women, passing through our village with the herds, warned my mother to start mourning me. Children rarely survived the malady to which I had succumbed—common enough in the village, but not so well known in the wider world as to have a European name. None of the western drugs that my parents had stockpiled for emergencies had any effect on my violent symptoms, and we were hundreds of miles from any biomedical facility. In the end, our wonderful neighbour Gudé insisted on calling in the local healer, a practitioner of classical Islamic medicine (mingled perhaps with some of the more persistent local practices). He carefully listened to her description of my case (my mother's Hausa, Gudé determined, was insufficient for life or death situations). Then he ground together an inky black—and memorably foul-tasting—tonic, and I drank it. I lived.

The second encounter took place a few years later, back in Massachusetts. It began with a school nurse and a needle. Purely by chance, I was in the last cohort of Boston children to be routinely screened for tuberculosis at school age. To the amazement of the school nurse—who had not seen a reactor for years—my arm swelled like a football around the test site. Thus began a sequence of tests, x-rays, doctors' conferences, examinations by excited medical students, injections, and a nauseating regime of drugs that (to the horror of my classmates) made me cry bright orange tears, and develop spidery veins all over my cheeks. It was far from enjoyable, but it cured my tuberculosis. Two years later, I was fit, healthy, and possessed of an extensive medical vocabulary. Back in Nigeria, the woman who unknowingly infected me was not so lucky. She died of TB sometime during those same years, having almost certainly passed her illness on to the family she loved, as well as the little girl whom she spoiled with homemade treats at a glorious wedding feast.

Looking back on these events as a western adult and a trained historian, I could offer any number of biomedical reinterpretations of each episode. My sister and I were far better nourished than our village peers; in fact, as an 8 year-old, my sister was a tall as many girls of marriageable age (and her lucky blue eyes brought in at least one fine proposal from a passing Taureg trader). Our better overall health, rather than the bitter medicine, might explain why I survived what was so often a killer disease. Or perhaps the traditional remedy, tested empirically for generations, contained some powerful plant medicine: let the bioprospecting begin!

Meanwhile, it may seem self-evident that—however uncomfortable, however awkward they made school life—the scary side effects of my anti-TB treatment were worth enduring to ensure my speedy recovery, and the safety of my family and classmates. An earlier generation of western doctors, however, would by no means have agreed that the risks to which I was exposed by the powerful antibiotic chemotherapy were either necessary or worthwhile. As an otherwise healthy child in the early stages of disease, my tuberculosis could have been treated by a regime of nutrition and exercise designed to improve my general health and enable my own body to fight off the infection. The health of others could have been protected either by isolating me in a sanatorium, or by the implementation of rigorous hygienic discipline in my own home. Were those doctors just old-fashioned and resistant to change, or were they ahead of their time in advocating low-tech therapeutic methods that improved overall health and had no iatrogenic risks attached? As so often in medicine, there is no perfect treatment for TB. The older generation's solution to tuberculosis was certainly effective in many cases like my own, and of course had no adverse physical side effects. Tuberculosis could never become resistant to the sanatorium solution—but it was costly, disruptive of family life, and time-consuming. It also involved rather more exercise, fresh air, and sleeping outdoors in the cold than I personally would have welcomed.

I certainly have no regrets about being born in late twentieth-century North America, and no doubts about the power of biomedicine. I'm a big fan of antibiotics. But my own experiences showed me that biomedical knowledge is far from complete—remember, biomedicine did not even have a name for my village illness, much less a cure for it. As a disease affecting predominantly poor rural African children, it attracted the attention neither of colonial or post-colonial administrators (who focused their medical efforts on the workforce), nor of pharmaceutical entrepreneurs (who innovate first for those who can pay)—and in a Muslim region, there were few missionaries to publicize its tragic effects. I also know that our Islamic doctor was neither a quack nor a fool; like any western general practitioner, he knew that there were times to intervene actively and medically, and times to deploy non-medical forces, like those represented by a protective amulet.

As a child, it never occurred to me to question the expertise of my various medical practitioners, or the assumptions that underpinned their different modes of therapy. As an adult, I may have found occasion to doubt the former, and as a scholar, I am professionally trained to inter-rogate the latter—but having been successfully healed in two very different medical cultures, I am constitutionally unable to privilege any particular one monolithically. 'Medicine' in any culture comprises be-liefs as well as facts, experiences as well as knowledge, expectations as well as effects. It is an interpretive as well as a descriptive and prescriptive discipline. As such, the persistence and success of a medical system is invariably contingent not only on its therapeutic efficacy, but on the historical and cultural climate within which it operates and to which it responds. Thus in this book, I will examine medical systems from several global cultures—the Introduction will set the stage by describing and comparing classical and modern western medicine, Ayurveda, and Chinese medicine—and consider their interactions over four centuries.

Those four centuries, from the seventeenth through the twenti-eth, were in many ways transformative both of western medicine and of the western and non-western worlds. (Although it will not be a major theme of this book, this period was no less transformative of non-western medicine. References and further reading on this subject will be suggested at the end of the book.) Through com-parisons between different medical innovations and importations across the entire period, each chapter will further explore the twin processes of medical and historical change through the eyes of the medical professionals and consumers of the day. In Chapter 1, I'll tell the familiar story of customer dissatisfaction with established medicine—and desperate self-experimentation—in rather less familiar places: late seventeenth-century Indonesia and later the

Low Countries and Britain. And even to twenty-first-century consumers, the remedies involved are pretty exotic: acupuncture and moxabustion. A century later, despite rapid advances in medical and natural knowledge, Western European patients remained sceptical of the increasingly powerful medical profession and its monopolistic claims. Chapter 2 examines this period, and the rise of two genuinely 'alternative' European medical systems: homeopathy and mesmerism. Chapter 3 looks again at acupuncture, this time in the nineteenth century, when it was one of the first surgical techniques to be tested by scientific experiment. The chapter also compares professional and consumer attitudes towards acupuncture and homeopathy, exposing both similarities and differences between our responses to medical innovations from within our own culture and from other cultures. Chapter 4 moves away from the western world, to look at the historical impact of cross-cultural medical exchanges in non-western contexts. Not every medical culture has been as suspicious of, or as antagonistic to, other medicines as has been western medicine. Yet even in highly pluralistic cultures like that of India, history and politics played major roles in the ways in which non-indigenous medical innovations were received. To look at the relative importance of both historical context, and cultural attitudes towards 'multicultural medicine', I examine responses to two 'alternative' medicines (homeopathy and mesmerism) and one staple of mainstream western medicine (germ theory) in India, discovering in the process why a Scottish doctor might call himself a conjuror, and the ground shared by Ayurveda and quantum physics. Finally, the Conclusion considers the global medicine with which we live today. From Tiger Balm to 'Ayurvedic' skincare, consumers today can choose from an ever more diverse range of products and therapies. Perhaps even more importantly, they can learn about other medical cultures more easily and in more ways than ever before. But does that make our current fascination with exotic cures different from the fads and fancies of our predecessors? This closing chapter describes both the continuities and the distinctiveness of contemporary medical globalism.

ACKNOWLEDGEMENTS

A book like this—looking at different cultures over several centuries—necessarily depends heavily on the work of others. Throughout the volume, the scholars on whom I draw are cited; to some, however, I owe additional thanks. David Arnold not only wrote the pioneering studies of medicine in colonial India on which I've built my argument, but generously read through the relevant chapters, correcting my more egregious errors. Long ago and far away, Dominik Wujastik and Kan-Wen Ma did me the same favour on earlier versions of my material on Indian and Chinese medical systems. To all three of these more erudite scholars I am enormously grateful; any remaining flaws are, of course, entirely of my own introduction. To Philip Nicholls and Alison Winter, too, I am indebted. Their work on, respectively, homeopathy and mesmerism was invaluable. No historian of medicine or medical culture, particularly in the Enlightenment, can fail to lean on the late Roy Porter, but I was unusually fortunate in having him for a mentor. In 1997, he told me to write a book on alternative medicine—I am sure he would laugh at how long it has taken me to follow his advice. Around the same time, Londa Schiebinger reminded me that a good book was worth taking time over. I may have taken these words a bit too literally, but along with her body of work, they inspired me to keep slogging away. My 'writing buddy' Ian Burney gave me much insight and support, and a great excuse for productive coffee breaks, as did other colleagues at the Universities of Manchester and Houston, not least John Pickstone, Roger Cooter, Marty Melosi, Eric Walther, and Joe Pratt. Chandak Sengoopta finished his book and proved it was possible. Nevertheless, without Rima Apple, I would never have finished mine. Her encouragement, her warmth, and especially her stern questions about its progress were inspirational. Grants from the Wellcome Trust and the University of Houston supported my work on this volume, and the Wellcome Library, along with Harvard's Widener and the British Library, were homes from home while I researched it.

Many students shaped this volume. Some, however, did much more than their fair share. I would like to express my gratitude to the University of Houston students who read and laughed and questioned their way through 3303 Medicine in America, 3394 Medicine and Empire, and 3394 Encountering Illness. They tackled huge questions and hard readings, often with frustratingly little background or preparation. I knew they could do it—but they did it so well! And then nagged me to do my part better. I hope this book answers all those questions I said we could come back to . . .

As well as these professional debts, I have personal thanks to give. My family has supported me throughout this project—and since my progress was slow and painful, they put up with more than their fair share of long silences and grumbling, for which tolerance I am deeply grateful. The Ettrick family, too, was generous, and more than patient as I covered their beautiful home with crumpled pages. Helen Valier made my prose more readable, and made Chapters 2 and 3 possible at all: without her encouragement, I would never have survived even homeopathic doses of them. Dominique Tobbell was another stalwart, reading far too many chapters whilst fibbing that it was no trouble (I didn't believe her—but I sent the chapters anyway). Hannah and Chris heard my woes and cheered me on over many a Texan brunch. John and Toni, Kate and Ben welcomed me back to Britain; and Keir, Bill, and Val helped me settle into Wales, making the last stage of this book far more pleasant than it would otherwise have been. Betty, Carolyn, Julie, and Claudia kept me sane, as always, when hysteria set in. Lisa came in, just at the end—and made getting it done worthwhile.

REB

CONTENTS

LIST OF ILLUSTRATIONS

ILLUSTRATION CREDITS

Courtesy of the US National Library of Medicine: 5, 8, 19, 21; courtesy of the William H. Helfand Collection, New York: 20; The Wellcome Library, London: 1, 2, 3, 4, 6, 7, 9, 10, 11, 12, 13, 14, 15, 16, 17, 18, 23, 24.

INTRODUCTION: 'RIVAL SYSTEMS OF MEDICINE'?

Walk into your local health food shop, café, or pick up the local paper. Chances are that you'll see ads for meditation, acupuncture, herbal supplements, and T'ai Chi classes, alongside the business cards of homeopaths and naturopaths, faith healers and Chinese herbalists. Prominent medical and scientific journals begrudge what they see as ill-considered enthusiasm for such 'heterodox' or 'alternative' therapies, and mourn the lost lustre of orthodox medicine.[1] Many orthodox practitioners berate patients for their 'flight from reason', while a smaller group adopts aspects or styles of alternative practice themselves. And indeed, since the 1970s, there has been an extraordinary rise in the availability and visibility of 'alternative', 'complementary', and 'cross-cultural' medicines. But is the astonishing popularity of heterodox medicine novel? Certainly, there have been other periods of tumultuous competition between medical systems, periods that powerfully shaped today's biomedicine. Bodily health and corporeal beauty have deep significance in historical, as well as contemporary, western cultures, and biomedicine has never been alone in seeking to provide them to an eager public. Consider the case of R.B., businessman, gentleman about town, and medical consumer.

In May 1836, R.B. was walking along the Strand in London when he spotted an intriguing headline in one of the capital's more controversial weeklies, a medical magazine called the *Lancet*. It described the successful use of a new and rather exotic medical technique to cure 'hydrocele' (a then common medical condition characterized by excessive fluid swelling of the scrotum). Our City gent was himself afflicted with hydrocele—hence his interest in the headline—and had recently consulted 'one of the most celebrated professors of surgery' about his condition. This consultation had left R.B. unimpressed by the proposed method of cure, an injection of port wine into the scrotum, which necessitated the loss of seven or eight working days in recovery time. Like many patients both then and now, he had therefore done nothing, perhaps hoping the problem would resolve itself. But the headline's claims stirred him to action: according to the *Lancet*'s report, his condition could be cured safely without invasive or painful therapies, with little or no inconvenience, and most importantly, without risking his testicles. He simply needed to submit to 'acupuncture'—described by the article as merely a few simple needle pricks. This 'operation' was much more to his taste:

I purchased the *Lancet* of May 7 [in which this technique was described], provided myself with a very fine needle and one of a larger size, and proceeded to puncture the lower end of the scrotum . . . After two insertions of the fine needle, without any apparent effect, I took the larger one. On its withdrawal an [*sic*] single drop of clear fluid followed. I endeavoured then, by pressure to force more, but could not succeed. . . . I abandoned the operation in despair of doing any good.[2]

Although apparently ineffective, the 'acupuncture' had at least fulfilled its promise of painlessness; he took a brisk walk and went home as usual. There, he discovered that he had despaired too soon: 'When undressing myself to go to bed, I found to my astonishment that *the whole of the swelling was reduced* . . . and this too without any other effusion of liquid.' He immediately sent a description of his success to the *Lancet*, and his letter appeared in a subsequent issue. From the *Lancet*, it was extracted and transmitted halfway around the world, to be reprinted by the *Journal of the Calcutta Medical and Physical Society* six months later in their regular column 'Spirit of the British Periodicals'.

What does this story offer to contemporary readers and medical inquirers? First, it illustrates the vital point that the cross-cultural transmission of medical knowledge and expertise—even 'alternative' medical knowledge and expertise—is not a uniquely contemporary phenomenon. Neither, evidently, was it ever a unidirectional process. The account documents a British response to a Chinese medical procedure, and the re-exportation of knowledge about that procedure to Britain's colonies in India. Second, it demonstrates a remarkable (at least to us) level of lay access to and participation in the medical press and the process of medical innovation. Not only was our businessman able to skim the *Lancet*'s headlines casually while perambulating on the Strand; he felt perfectly competent to buy it, read the article that had caught his eye, and perform the novel operation it described on his own body. Moreover, in 1836, our intrepid self-experimentalist could safely assume that the medical profession would be interested in his results and personal assessment of the medical innovation in question, despite his lay status. It is almost impossible to imagine a similar situation occurring today.

In demonstrating these two points, the story presents a surprising counterpoint to established views of both medical transmission and the patient role: clearly such transmission was neither unidirectional (from the western to the non-western world), nor restricted to the 'fringes' of medical culture. Clearly too, patients played active roles in the reception and integration of medical knowledge from other cultures, as in other areas of medical innovation. On the other hand, R.B.'s medical agnosticism is strikingly familiar. He was not opposed to orthodox medicine; indeed, he actively sought out a professional medical diagnosis and advice. However, he was also clearly willing to look beyond the established borders of orthodoxy—and even culture—for a cure. Thus, this article also serves as a useful reminder that the debates that characterize medicine today often reiterate historical arguments. Patients, practitioners, and medical policy-makers have encountered medical globalism and pluralism before, have fiercely contested the terrain of medical authority and orthodoxy, and have constantly relocated the balance of power in the doctor–patient relationship. By examining historical responses to alternative and cross-cultural medicine, we gain insight into the contemporary debate, and into the nature and effects of medical orthodoxy and heterodoxy alike. This volume will also explore the climates—medical, political, and cultural—in which 'cross-cultural' and 'alternative' medicines have flourished; and the ways in which these two often-undifferentiated categories are distinct from each other.

From a western and twentieth-first-century perspective, twentieth-century orthodox medicine—which I will call, for reasons of expediency, 'biomedicine'—looks both powerful and long-established.[3] It is apparently a monolithic system, holding a monopoly supported by a potent combination of laws, regulations, state and commercial interests, cultural beliefs and popular expectations. Biomedicine claims unique, exclusive, and absolute knowledge about the body in sickness and health, knowledge that is universally valid and ostensibly independent of cultural or social constraints or meaning. As a society, we accept these claims largely because we believe that biomedical knowledge is based on rigorous and objective scientific investigation of the natural world. Yet the sweeping cultural authority currently granted to science is, in historical terms, fairly new. As late as the eighteenth century, organized science was a target for the broadest of satires, and the subject of widespread scepticism.[4] Indeed, Jonathan Swift devoted the third volume of his famous *Gulliver's Travels* to a critique of the new Royal Society and of modern 'natural philosophy' in general. In 'A Voyage to Laputa', he depicts a society devoted to abstract thought, and governed in accordance with scientific principles rather than traditional values or even common sense. Of its elites, natural philosophers all, he wrote:

[A]lthough they were dextrous enough upon a Piece of Paper in the Management of the Rule, the Pencil, and the Divider, yet in the common Actions and Behaviour of Life, I have never seen a more clumsy, awkward and unhandy People, nor so slow and perplexed in their Conceptions upon all other Subjects, except those of Mathematicks and Musick. They are very bad Reasoners, and vehemently given to Opposition, unless when they happen to be of the right Opinion, which is seldom their case. . . . The whole Compass of their Thoughts and Mind [is] shut up within the forementioned Sciences.[5]

Still worse, these hapless elites have infected Lagodo, the mainland country under their governance, and laid it waste—all in the name of science/progress:

[A]bout forty years ago, certain persons went up to Laputa [the floating island home of the kingdom's leaders], . . . and after five months continuance, came back with very little smattering in Mathematicks, but full of the Volatile

Spirits acquired in that Airy Region. That these Persons upon their Return, began to dislike the Management of every Thing below; and fell into Schemes of putting all Arts, Sciences, Languages, and Mechanicks upon a new Foot. . . . The only Inconvenience is, that none of these Projects are yet brought to Perfection; and in the mean time, the whole Country lies miserably waste, the House in Ruins, and the People without Food or Cloaths. By all of which, instead of being discouraged, they are Fifty Times more violently bent on prosecuting their Schemes, driven on equally by Hope and Despair.[6]

In another part of the same Voyage, Swift narrates a visit to an island of sorcerers who can call up the spirits of the dead. His protagonist seizes this unique opportunity to pit champions of the Ancients and the Moderns against each other in supernatural debate. Needless to say, given Swift's strong ties to the Ancient cause, the proponents of science come out very much the losers. After comparing figures like Descartes, Gassendi, and Newton to Aristotle—and dismissing Newtonian gravity as a fad—Swift (speaking through the mouth of Aristotle's shade) asserted: 'the new Systems of Nature were but new Fashions, which would vary in every Age; and even those who pretend to demonstrate them from Mathematical Principles, would flourish but a short Period of Time, and be out of Vogue when that was determined'.[7]

Swift's irony is perhaps trumped by the fact that many of his air-castles and outrageous speculations—a system of 'scientific' agriculture in which 'all the Fruits of the Earth shall come to Maturity at whatever Season we think fit to chuse', for example—have become mundane reality and established fact in the centuries since he published *Gulliver's Travels*.[8] Nor was his unadulterated hostility to the new experimentally produced 'Systems of Nature' universally shared by his contemporaries. However, Swift's sense that abstract science had little to do with real life, and offered few practical benefits was common in the period—and indeed is not unknown today. He firmly believed that science and the Baconian 'scientific method' were merely faddish, and rejected outright the idea that knowledge created through experiment was better or more accurate that knowledge rooted in experience or (ancient) precedent. Swift's views reflected those of many physicians in his own time and well into the twentieth century.

As in Laputa, supporters of the scientific endeavour in the non-fictional realms of Western Europe had relatively little of practical utility to show for their efforts in the early years of the eighteenth century. In medicine, increasing interest in anatomy and dissection would not produce practical benefits to the sick patient for decades to come. Doctors and other healers continued to use the humours as their primary explanatory mode, as did their patients. But their inability to produce cures, despite their claims to ever more knowledge of the body's inner workings, left patients dissatisfied and in many cases disgusted.

Perhaps in part because of our perceptions of such medical inefficacy, the eighteenth century has been frequently described as the Golden Age of quackery; certainly, it saw a great flowering of medical commercialism and ingenuity, and luxuriant growth in the medical marketplace. What it did not possess in any great measure were any identifiable alternative medicines 'because there was no defined medical establishment against which they could react'.[9] Quacks, as Roy Porter has comprehensively demonstrated, did not present their medicines or therapies as 'alternative' to those of orthodox physicians, apothecaries, or surgeons, but as *better*. They did not propose different medical systems or models of the body, or even different understandings of diseases, but argued that their remedies operated more effectively than their competitors, under the same 'rules'. And what were those rules? Until the closing years of the century, the rules of health followed by patients and practitioners alike were largely unchanged from those reborn with the Renaissance reappraisal of Galen (CE 130-200) and the Reformation rediscovery of Hippocrates (circa 460–380 BCE).

Shared Boundaries: Medical Systems before 'Scientific Medicine'

Imagine a world in which your health depended not just on your own actions or inactions—what you ate or drank, how long you slept, your sexual activity, your level of exposure to healthy or

DE ASTROLOGIA

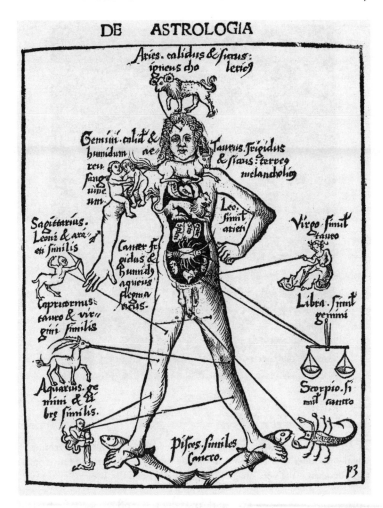

1. 'Astrological man' from Gregor Reisch, *Margarita Philosophica*, c.1503. Note that specific areas or organs of the body are associated with particular astrological signs, and that the signs themselves are linked to particular humoural traits and temperaments. Compare this to Chinese Five Elements theory.

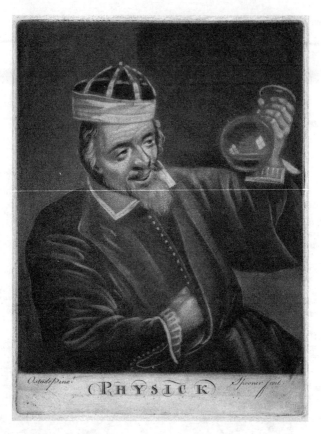

Ostade pinx.   (PHYSICK)   *Spooner fecit*

2. A physician examining a flask of urine, seventeenth-century mezzotint by Charles Spooner after Adriaen van Ostade. In his velvet cap and fine clothes, this physician is the very image of scholarly physic in the West.

unhealthy environments, and the degree and types of physical exertion demanded by your daily life—but on the seasons, the weather, the exact nature of your social interactions, and the motions of the heavens at the time of your birth and during any medical encounter. In this medical culture, elite healers are not marked out by their hands-on knowledge of human anatomy or physiology. Rather, the 'verrey parfit practisour' was one 'grounded in astronomye'; one who could tell the very hours of each patient's lifespan by 'magik naturel'.[10] They rarely, if ever, touch the bodies of their patients, diagnosing instead on the basis of astrological charts, visual examination of the patient's blood and urine, and close attention to the patient's spoken testimony and social position (see Figures 1 and 2). Surgery is only performed as a desperate last resort, since few survive its rigours and none opt for its agonies readily in a world without antiseptics and anaesthesia. Elite practitioners, moreover, scorn surgery's brutal and indecent familiarity with the body, and leave it in the hands of 'lesser'—or at least less educated and lower-class—healers (and there are many of these, trained and untrained, lay and professional, offering between them remedies to suit every budget and taste). Instead of such localized approaches to bodily ill health, most therapies are intended to heal through altering the entire corporeal system simultaneously. They consist of physical interventions like bleeding, purging, and vomiting; changes in diet and activity; and an array of highly complicated and expensive medical compounds, more mundane botanical simples, and some few 'specific' remedies for particular ailments (see Figures 3 and 4).

In this world, patients and healers share the conviction that bodily health depends on maintaining a precarious balance of the body's four constituent substances, or 'humours': materially, the humours can be seen in the blood, phlegm, black bile, and yellow bile. These substances can emerge spontaneously from the (sick) body, or be brought forth by medical or surgical interventions. They exist in a dynamic equilibrium with each other, with external influences like climate, seasons, and celestial spheres, and with internal forces like the ageing process and emotions (it is not coincidental that human temperaments here bear humoural names: choleric, melancholic, sanguine, and phlegmatic). Disturbances in health, whether of mind or body, simply reflect disturbances in humoural balance, and healers of every variety strive to diagnose such imbalances, and to redress them.

This medical culture, with its holistic links between mind, body, society, and environment, may seem very 'alternative' to twenty-first-century eyes. Its four 'humours' may likewise seem quaintly simple to readers who know their bodies as factories of innumerable

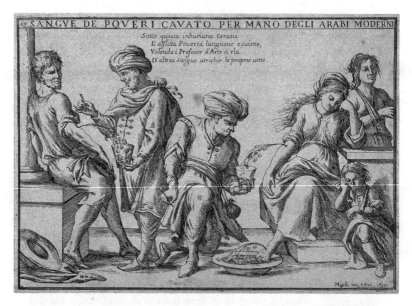

3. 'Sangue de poveri cavato par mano degli arabi moderni', Giuseppe Mitelli, 1699. At one level, this image illustrates the mechanics of bleeding—in its simplest form, practitioners simply opened a vein, catching the blood in a basin until the desired amount had been removed. But it also illustrates the persistent hostility with which western medical observers and commentators have received medical experts from other cultures. Arabic doctors are shown bleeding the Italian poor dry, as gold jets out of their veins with their blood.

active fluids orchestrating multiple organ systems, and designed to maintain stability in the face of drastic environmental shifts. Indeed, westerners may glimpse a resemblance between this healing system and those conventionally associated with the non-western world. Yet the medical world I have depicted is that of Western Europe for much of its history—from the classical period until at least the end of the eighteenth century. It is the world of Hippocrates, still celebrated as the 'father of western medicine' even today. If orthodoxy in medicine is in part determined by the durability and degree of acceptance achieved by any particular medical idea, then this picture—though to us strange and exotic—is a portrait of 'orthodox

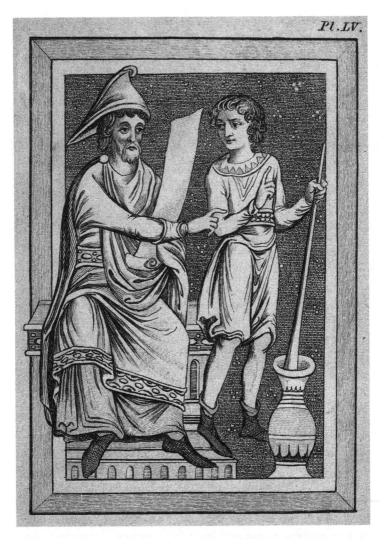

Pl. LV.

4. Physician reading a complex recipe while his assistant prepares ingredients using mortar and pestle, engraving based on twelfth-century manuscript.

western medicine'. It certainly endured unchallenged for far longer than biomedicine, a mere upstart with a scant century of widespread use and acceptance to its credit. Indeed, some argue that 'humouralism' (as this system is known) still informs our day-to-day conceptions of health and disease: 'feed a cold and starve a fever'; 'you'll catch your death of cold'; 'a shock to the system'—all are phrases which draw their meaning from the ancient humoural model. Moreover, biomedicine itself has been seriously challenged from its inception by medical systems that draw much of their persuasive force from their attention to the whole patient, and their reliance on humoural modes of explanation.

Among the most prominent challengers to biomedical orthodoxy today, for reasons that I will examine in later chapters, are practices that originated in South and East Asia. They seem to have little in common with biomedicine, and many critics have argued that it is their difference (rather than any particular efficacy, or medical merit) that renders them so attractive. Medical alternatives with European and North American origins—for instance, homeopathy, mesmerism (now often called medical hypnotism), and naturopathy—seem equally distant, both in their underlying theories and in their methods, from today's medical mainstream. But it is well worth considering that until quite recently, all secular healers and medical systems, whatever their claims to 'orthodoxy', operated within a common set of limits: none had any route of direct access to the internal workings of the body, because there was no way to safely open living bodies and look inside. Rather, internal functions and systems had to be inferred from a narrow range of indirect evidence. Bodily function or malfunction could be assessed in part by the body's intake and output—by what individuals craved, ate, and drank; by the patterns of their respirations; and by the rate, type, and appearance of their excretions (sweat, mucus, urine, faeces, vomit, and for women, menstrual blood). And there were a few windows to the interior: blood could be taken and examined by sight and taste; the heartbeat and breathing could be heard through the body's walls; the whites of the eyes, the coating of the tongue, and the colour of the complexion were available for visual analysis; touch could reveal a certain amount about the body's temperature; and both the body and breath had characteristic odours and tastes in certain conditions. Moreover, individuals did (and of course still do) have direct access to their own bodily sensations and experience, and could provide vital—but not necessarily accurate, complete, or intelligible—information about the body's invisible interior. Finally, healers around the world opportunistically studied the body's cavities and viscera when chance (and war) made them available, and many cultures also dissected animals and the occasional cadaver. These were, for all intents and purposes, the parameters of the diagnostic universe for healers of all stripes and every culture until the eighteenth and early nineteenth century.

Unsurprisingly, operating within these narrow confines, healers developed similar intellectual and material approaches to the body. Globally, perhaps the most common tenet of pre-modern medical practice is the idea that the human body is a microcosm of the universe (see Figure 5). Chinese, Indian, and European medical thinkers believed that the cosmos and the corporeal were composed of the same basic materials. This shared substance meant that the behaviour and relations of these building blocks in the greater cosmological world could define and predict their behaviour and relations in the smaller corporeal one. Thus, for example, Chinese thinkers recognized five 'elements' (or, more accurately, five types of processes, each of which was represented by an archetypal substance) in the natural world—metal, wood, water, fire, and earth. The Chinese macrocosm correspondingly contained five recognized planets, five climates, five compass directions (the Chinese included 'centre' as well as the cardinal directions), five tastes, and five smells. Since the human body mirrored in miniature this natural world, Chinese medicine was organized around five viscera—the heart, the liver, the spleen, the lungs, and the kidneys, each of which was also associated with a particular element (fire, wood, earth, metal, and water, respectively). As in the parallel cases of Europe and India, this particular constellation of organs was called into existence by the demands of cosmology (theories of the universe) as well as the evidence of experience, animal dissection, and chance observations

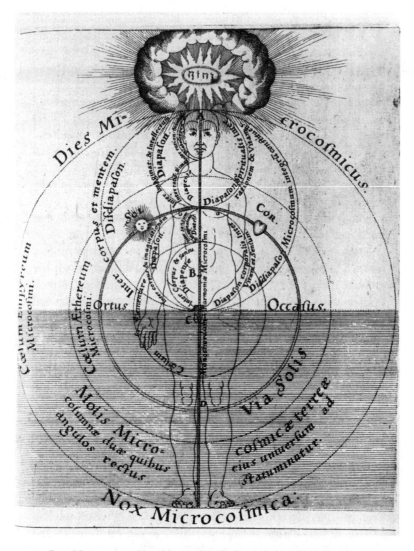

5. *Dies Microcosmicus: Nox Microcosmica*, Robert Fludd, 1617–18. A western alchemical chart, showing the human body as the world soul, and likening the heart to the sun (hinting at the circulation of the blood).

of human anatomy. The affinity of the organs to the elemental substances signified the likeness between the organs and the processes of which the different elements were emblematic. Each organ therefore also partook of the other attributes characteristic of the element/process with which it shared symbolic substance.

In the fully elaborated model of this corporeal universe developed by the Chinese, called 'Five Element theory', specific organs were associated with the odours, tastes, colours, sensations, emotions, seasons, planets, and even compass directions identified with the same element. This meant that every aspect of the natural environment that was available to the senses was also represented in the body, in one or another of the five viscera. The parallels between the Chinese system and its analogues in classical and medieval European medicine, and in India's Ayurvedic texts, are remarkable. European doctors likewise associated body parts and organs to particular seasons, star signs, and elements, and the five great Hindu elements are indivisible from aspects of the body and objects of the senses.

These intimate links between the body and the external world profoundly affected the ways in which healers and philosophers in each of these medical cultures understood sickness and health. Across all three medical systems, practitioners regarded disease to be a state of imbalance within the body, caused or perpetuated by disharmony in the interactions between individuals and their environment. The aim of all medical treatment was consequently to preserve or restore a healthy dynamic equilibrium both internally and externally. This was a task demanding vigilant and consistent effort on the part of both patients and healers. Diet, levels of activity and rest, and ageing all affected the state of the body, as did the weather, the changing seasons, and locality. Additionally, in Chinese and Indian medicine, and to an only slightly lesser degree, in western medicine, the healthful balance could be affected by changing states *either* of body or of mind—excesses of emotion might either cause bodily illness or be caused by it. Consciousness in classical Chinese medical theory (as in the most materialistic models of western medicine today, though for rather different reasons) was an organ of the body rather than a separate entity residing within it. The Ayurvedic canon likewise argued that while the mind creates the body, it is also dependent upon it. As one western commentator observed, in Indian medical thought, 'the soul can (with great difficulty) be extracted from the body, but then so (with much greater ease) may a heart or a tongue'.[11]

For western healers, these interactions between body and mind, and body and environment, were mediated by the humoural fluids. These fluids were produced by the different organs and circulated through the body. Their production was affected by the changing seasons and by the aspect of the planets with which each was associated, as well as by diet and physical or mental actions. Individuals were healthy only when their bodies achieved the humoural balance that was appropriate not only to their ages, temperaments, habits, and employments, but also to their environments. In Indian and Chinese medicine too, fluids imbued with unique properties and actions and capable of affecting the physical and mental state of the body mediated the relationship between the organs, the body, and the social and natural environments.

However, the broad parallels between these three 'scholarly' (in other words, learned, text-based, and systematically transmitted) medical traditions should not obscure the ways in which they differ from each other and from modern biomedicine. Differences— material, theoretical, and institutional—between subcontinental, East Asian, and western medical systems influenced their rates of transmission and styles of reception in the global medical marketplace at least as deeply as their similarities. The next two sections set out basic principles of subcontinental and East Asian medicine, and compare those systems to their western counterpart (referred to here for convenience as 'pre-modern' or 'scholastic' western medicine).

Medicine in India: Ayurveda, Siddha, and Unani Tibb

As with so much of India's culture, its indigenous medical practices have their roots in the ancient religious and philosophical writings called the *Vedas*—'the knowledge'.[12] These texts took their current form in the second millennium BCE. They describe the origins of the universe, the natural world, the human race, and the social order.

Perhaps more importantly, the Vedas set out the principles upon which Hindu religious, moral, and social life is based. In the process, they paint a fragmented but fascinating picture of an understanding of health and the body based on religious and magical principles, but also upon direct and careful observation of natural events.

The first group of specifically therapeutic ideas emerged at around the time of the Buddha (*c.*450 BCE), and were transcribed and codified thereafter, taking their current form as compilations (samhitas) in the first centuries of the Common Era. While these works explicitly root themselves in the Vedic tradition, they also clearly draw on the learning of heterodox groups like the Buddhists and Jains, and on the writings of individual ascetics—pluralism can therefore be regarded as an integral and formative aspect part of the medical culture of the subcontinent. Even the body in Ayurvedic medicine is represented by two somewhat different models. One looks quite familiar to western eyes: it envisions the body as a system composed of ducts and tubes, valves and burners (see Figure 6). It is very similar to the hydraulic model that became popular in late seventeenth-century Europe as the workings of the circulatory system came to be known. Like the hydraulic model, this Indian body is the product of centuries of careful, empirical observations (filtered, as in the West, through an elaborate medical cosmology), and offers straightforward answers to most of the 'how' and 'what' questions in medicine: 'How do the humours flow around the body?' 'What makes the body warm?'

A Tamil variant of Ayurveda called Siddha medicine, meanwhile, offered another way of thinking about the body and its functions, portraying it as an alchemical laboratory. The healthy body takes in gross matter and purifies it through the metabolic processes of digestion and circulation. The component of spirit or energy which exists in every natural object, and which is identical with the life force, is thus released to the body. This alchemical body explains the functions of bodily processes, and seems to have arisen as a way to address medical 'why' and more complex 'how' questions: 'Why do humans eat and excrete?' 'Why do people fall ill?' 'How does the weather affect health?' It is also linked to deeper philosophical and

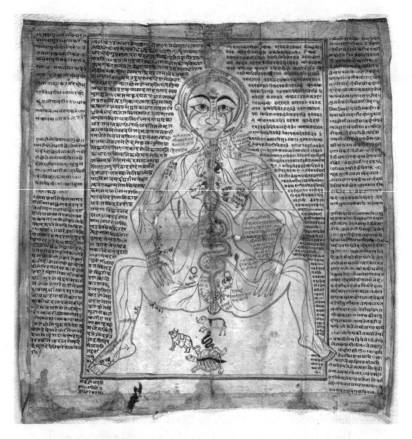

6. Ayurvedic tantric (alchemical) body, taken from an eighteenth-century manuscript, and illustrating the flow of *prana* (the life force) through the body. Intriguingly, the image closely resembles late fourteenth-century Persian anatomical drawings.

cosmological inquiries by the spiritual alchemy of reincarnation and karma. Just as the body acts to free spirit, or *ojas*, from gross matter, so embodiment over the course of many life cycles acts to purify the individual soul (or 'atman') of its worldly attachments and free it from slavery to matter. In Vagbhata's *Heart of Medicine* (written *c.*600 CE) *ojas* is described in some detail:

It is said, however, that the ultimate power in all the body tissues, right up to seed, is *ojas*. Although it is based in the heart, it permeates, maintaining the continuity of the body. It is unctuous . . . pure, and slightly reddish yellow. When it goes, one is lost; when it stays, one survives. It is that from which the various states present in the body arise. The things that make *ojas* decrease are: anger, hunger, worry, grief, fatigue and the like . . . But when the *ojas* increases, one's body feels well, properly nourished, and strong.

This combination of material and immaterial characteristic suggests that another appropriate translation for *ojas* in the corporeal (as opposed to the ethereal) body is 'energy', or 'vital energy'. Medically, the idea that such an important bodily constituent was affected by the events, choices, and actions of past lives explained otherwise inexplicable health or illness. In each of these visions of the body, balanced and healthy interactions with the environment are essential, not just for the body itself, but for the soul.

These models explain the physical phenomena of health and illness in Ayurvedic medicine. In both, the physical body is constituted by seven tissues—*dhatu* in Sanskrit. These tissues bind mind and spirit to the physical body, while strengthening and supporting them. Ayurveda's parallel to the western humours (*dosa* in Sanskrit) circulate around the *dhatus*. These vital fluids are *vata*, *pitta*, and *kapha*—wind or breath, bile, and phlegm—and as in western humouralism, they are considered to be physical substances. But medically the *dosas* differ from the humours in that they are not treated as purely physical fluids. Simultaneously, they represent the active elements—air (paired with space), fire (paired with water), and water (paired with earth)—in Ayurveda's alchemical body-model, and thus are linked to the attributes and affinities of those elements. One further association unites their alchemical and hydraulic roles: they are the less stable, more impure forms of the vital essences, *agni*, *prana*, and *ojas*—understood as the forms in which the elements of air, fire and water exist in living beings.

A third system of medicine became widespread on the subcontinent after the Muslim conquests of the eleventh century, and was strengthened by the rise of the Mughal Empire in the sixteenth century. Called *Unani* (an indigenous transliteration of the Greek 'Ionian') *Tibb*, it was introduced and practised primarily by Muslims and would come to be closely identified with South Asian Islam by the end of the nineteenth century. However, like western scholastic medicine, Unani Tibb originated in the medical thought and treatises of the classical world. It was based on the four Galenic humours, and shares with western medicine the Galenic model of a tripartite functional body, composed of vegetative, animal, and rational 'souls', joined to operate on the *pneuma* (air' or vital spirit) to sustain both physical and spiritual life. However, Islamic medicine in this period was highly cosmopolitan, drawing also on the medical traditions of the entire Islamic world, from North Africa to the Iberian Peninsula to the subcontinent itself. Like all of India's medical systems (and like the prevailing medical systems in East Asia and Europe), Unani Tibb incorporated astrology and prayer with more materialist pharmaceutics, hydraulic and alchemical notions of the body, and much close and astute observation of the processes of sickness and health. Because of its substantial overlap with pre-modern western medicine, Unani Tibb will not be discussed separately here.

Medicine in East Asia: Five Elements, Twelve Rivers, and the 'Return to the Void'

The connections made in East Asian medicine between cosmology and the natural world—including the human body—are similar in many respects to Ayurveda. As with Ayurveda, much of East Asian medical theory emerges from a more ancient narrative of the creation of the universe and of the natural world. This story, like that of the Vedas (with which it is roughly contemporary), combines an overarching belief in the unity of nature with a group of nested ordering categories, into one of which all natural objects must fall. These categories are themselves defined through a set of material traits and characteristics. The first recorded traces of this system (familiar to westerners through the terms *yin* and *yang*, its two primary sub-categories) develop lines of correspondence or association between sets of theoretically opposed states of being, characteristics, and physical phenomena. Thus, the attributes 'feminine' and 'masculine' are linked to similarly opposed physical phenomena lllike, respectively, dark and light, wet and dry, cold and warm. All of the first terms were associated with the category *yin*, and all the latter with its opposite term, *yang*.[13] Intriguingly, many of the pairings of opposed characteristics are exactly duplicated within western medical thought, particularly those that associate the feminine with passivity, coldness, wetness, and other negatively charged states. East Asian medical thought differs from its western analogue, however, in that it does not impose a rigid duality or expect a binary division of traits. Instead, it stresses that within each predominantly yin or yang entity, characteristics associated with its opposite occur; nothing is pure yin or pure yang (see Table 1).

The earliest surviving medical text, the *Huangdi Neijing* (or *Yellow Emperor's Inner Canon*), written *c*.200 BCE depends on and develops this system of yin/yang correspondence, as well as the Five Element theory which is its counterpoint. Like the Ayurvedic medical texts, the *Neijing* considers the human body as a microcosm of the universe—but as seen from a Chinese perspective. This vision of the body therefore reflected in minute detail the state, culture, and even the physical landscape within which it was written (see Figure 7). The body was a tiny country, with a ruler, eleven other state officials, ministers, and assistants working harmoniously to run the vital transport and communication systems. Within the body, both of these functions took place via twelve waterways (*jing*)— reflecting the macrocosmic twelve great rivers and canals of China—and ever-smaller sub-channels called *luo* and *sun*, as well as vessels called *mai*, located in vital regions of the body. Through each of these channels flowed a fluid substance called *qi* (the *mai* also transported blood). All along the channels were points or depots called *xue*, where the flow of *qi* was accessible to outside (medical) influences. These channels connected the organs to each other and also allowed each internal organ to communicate with a surface 'organ' (for example, the liver connects with the eyes) an idea that became essential to diagnosis. This model of the body represents the *Huangdi Neijing*'s major theoretical contribution to East Asian medical thought. Otherwise, the text focuses pragmatically on descriptions

TABLE I

	Yin	Yang
General Qualities	feminine, earth	masculine, heavens
	dark, cold, wet	light, hot, dry
In the body	the lower parts and front, the inner parts and deeper organs, and the solid organs are relatively more yin	the upper parts and back, the outer parts (e.g. hair, skin), the shallower organs; the hollow organs are all relatively more yang
Organs	yin organs are those which produce, regulate, transform, and store the fundamental-substances: *qi* (essence or energy producing movement) blood, *jing* (essence or energy producing organic develop-ment), *shen* (spirit, material consciousness), fluids (bodily juices)	yang organs are those which receive, break down, and absorb that part of the food that will become fundamental substances; they also transport and excrete the rest
Characteris-tic illness	dampness	heat
Pernicious influence	here, the atmospheric condition of dampness has invaded a body imbalanced by excess yin energy. Symp-toms include heavy mucoid secretion and discharges, oozing skin—typical western diagnosis might include herpes zoster, other viral infections	here, the atmospheric condition of heat has invaded a body imbalanced by excess yang energy. Symptoms include sudden fevers and hot rashes—typical western diagnosis might be a bacterial infection, like Streptococcus
Therapies	herbal treatments, as their effects are produced through digestion (and thus move from interior to exterior)	acupuncture and moxabustion because they move from exterior to interior

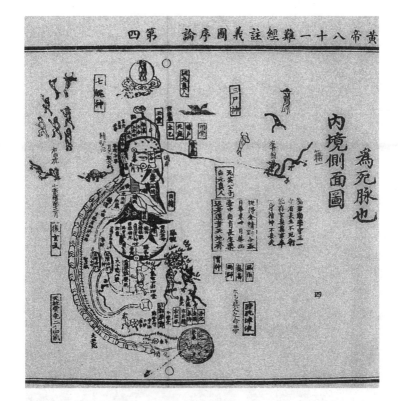

7. 'Illustration of internal topography [*neijing*], side view', from the *Canon of Eighty-One Problems of the Yellow Lord with Illustrations and Exegesis*, fifteenth-century Chinese woodblock illustrating the inner world of the human body in Daoist philosophy. Note the rivers, canals, and depots, so similar to those of China's countryside. The body image is surrounded by drawings hinting at Daoist practices of internal alchemy (directed at achieving hyper-longevity).

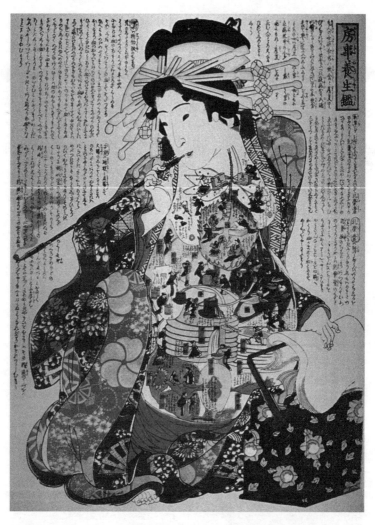

8. 'Woman smoking a pipe', nineteenth-century Japanese poster. This image vividly depicts the idea of the human body as a microcosm of the world as it flourished in an Asian context: bodily processes are illustrated by pictures of daily village life: people work at little machines, till and harvest in fields, and appear to speak and pray. The woman may be pregnant, as there is a shadow in her womb. Compare with Illustration 7, a much earlier Chinese version of the same concepts.

of diseases and their therapies, and on praising preventive medicine. The latter emphasis illustrates the traditional view in Chinese medicine that the good doctor maintains the health of his or her patients, and thus does not need to perform miraculous cures.

As in the Ayurvedic and humoural models of the body and its organs, each Chinese organ was associated with one of the archetypal substances, and with all of its linked qualities and affinities. Like Ayurveda, Chinese medicine has traditionally been concerned with functional rather than structural anatomy—in other words, Chinese doctors focused on physiology (which, of course, could be assessed from the outside) rather than on physical structure (which would have demanded extensive, and culturally forbidden dissection). Thus, despite sharing names with the western anatomical organs, the 'organs' in Chinese anatomy should be considered not as physical entities but as groups of closely related physiological functions. As well as elucidating this functionalist approach to anatomy, early Chinese texts also define the principle fluid components of the body: the Fundamental Substances. Like their analogues in Ayurvedic medicine and Galenic humouralism, these follow a hierarchy from more to less crudely material. Many—including blood, sweat, saliva, and the gastric fluids—are extracted at greater or lesser degrees of refinement directly from food. Others, particularly *jing, qi*, and *shen* (collectively known as the San Bao or 'three gems' for their importance to health and well-being) are far more complex substances. *Jing* is the natural energy or strength that the body derives from food. *Jing* is refined into *qi*; together, these substances allow the body to grow and develop, and supply its capacity to act. *Shen,* unlike *jing* and *qi,* is unique to human life and is the substance that enables awareness. The traditional formula for expressing the relationship that these substances have to one another is strongly reminiscent of Ayurvedic ideas and both Siddha and European alchemy: 'Refine the *jing* to transform the *qi*, refine the *qi* to transform the *shen*, refine the *shen* and return to the void,' although western alchemical formulations focused on purification as a tool to gain access to the divine, rather than as a means by which to reunite with the primal void.[14] All three of these substances were regarded as essential to life, but although without *shen* the body dies, it plays a comparatively small role in medical practice. *Qi* and *jing* are more accessible to human and medical intervention.

As in Ayurvedic and western medicine, the subtle fluids—and in particular, *qi*—act as the mediators between body, mind and environment. The maintenance of a healthy balance between the different organs, and all of the qualities and attributes which they represent, depends fundamentally on a free circulation of *qi*. *Ojas* (spirit or energy) is a close analogue of *qi* in Indian medicine, while the *aether* or *pneuma* of the ancient Greeks and the *spiritus animalis* of Galen fulfil the same roles in the West. Like these substances in their own milieux, *qi* takes many forms and natures in Chinese philosophy. The word itself, like its Greek analogue *pneuma*, is polysemic. It can refer to the literal breath, to wind in the meteorological sense, and to the universal vital principle, as well as to the body's life force or vital energy. The form of *qi* which circulates around, nourishes, and protects the organs is sometimes specified in the Chinese medical literature by the term *Zheng-qi* or 'proper breath'. This form of *qi* is particularly susceptible to human interventions—exercise, diet, medicine, and change of climate—and is therefore the most important in medical terms.

The conception of the body which underpins Indian, Chinese, and western scholastic medicine is one of a largely fluid entity in dynamic equilibrium, unified but permeable to environmental forces. These bodies interact, through perception and digestion, with the physical environment and the social structure; they are affected by and affect changing mental states. Religion too plays a role in each system, underpinning cosmological beliefs and offering an additional explanatory mode: supernatural as well as natural entities and actions could cause illness. For example in Ayurveda, the accumulated karma of the embodied soul (which, during its tenure in the body takes the form of *ojas*) can alter the body's health, and can explain illnesses not tractable to either alchemical or hydraulic explanations. In western medicine, prayer, repentance, and religious cleansing were resorts both of individuals and of societies in medical crises.

All of these bodies were endowed with vital energy, and were intercalated with consciousness through the senses or the emotions.

Thus the medical practices of these systems aim to augment, redirect, or restore the body's health-giving interactions with its mental, physical, and cultural surroundings. Therapies in South and East Asia in particular have been practically and theoretically designed to tap the vital healing energy and to restore its component substances, whether physical humours or subtle fluids like *qi* or *ojas*, to a proper state of dynamic balance. Indeed, the crucial role of the circulating subtle fluids in Ayurvedic and Chinese medicine illustrates one of the emerging differences between these systems and that of the West. In late seventeenth- and eighteenth-century Europe, the pulse was increasingly regarded as a merely two-dimensional indicator of bodily health; the western body-model placed far less emphasis on a complex circulation of subtle fluids than its Ayurvedic and Chinese counterparts so only quantifiable elements of the pulse—force and frequency—were significant. On the other hand, Ayurvedic and Chinese medicine—in which quasi-material, quasi-ethereal fluids like *qi* and *ojas* played vital roles in mediating relationships between internal organs—continued to depend heavily upon a multi-factorial pulse as a way to read the internal workings of the body.

Yin, yang, and the Five Phases in Chinese medicine; the Five Elements and three *Dosas* in Ayurveda; and the four humours in western humoural medicine play central roles in the diagnosis and treatment of disease in each medical system. The systems of correspondence constructed around these theories provide groups of physical, apparent clues to the hidden underlying characteristic and *systemic* condition of each patient. Thus, a pale woman with perpetually cold hands and feet, a pale tongue, and terrible menstrual cramps, could be readily diagnosed as a person with excess yin in China, while her cold, pallor, and problems in menstruation would suggest an excess of phlegm in the West, and *kapha* in India. Healers in each system could then gain deeper insight into the nature of the patient's complaint by further extending their exploration of cosmological correspondences. For example, the careful Chinese physician might try to determine for which of the Five Phases she had the greatest affinity: cold limbs would suggest Water, and if the patient had a foul, chemical odour, the association with Water would be confirmed. However, if she had a fragrant odour, it would suggest an affinity for Earth. The physician might also look for a failure in one of the organs. To do so, the practitioner would consider the relationship between the visible surface orifices or tissues (like the eyes, skin, or tongue) and their connected pairs of internal organs, as well as the Five Phases associations between organs and, for instance, emotions or seasons. Chinese diagnostics—and equally its Ayurvedic and humoural analogues—involved the active and empirical use of all of the senses, as well as detailed questioning of the patient. In combination with careful observation of each individual's demeanour, the patient's history could reveal any social and environmental factors relevant to disease.

By interpreting illness in terms of these more or less elaborate systems of correspondences, doctors added structure and analytical power to their empirical experience of disease. These three medical cosmologies also gave healers the intellectual tools they needed to recognize patterns, organize knowledge gained from experience, and render it more readily applicable. On the other hand, the multi-faceted complexity of the relationships between symptoms and correspondences preserved the diagnostic flexibility that was regarded as essential to dealing with the particular situation of individual patients. The combination of comprehensiveness, comprehensibility (these systems, after all, were not the exclusive property of medical communities, but embodied shared understandings of both macro- and microcosmic universe and its workings), and flexibility was a potent one. Indeed, Ayurveda and traditional Chinese medicine (TCM) continue to be practised in Europe and in their regions of origin today, and western humoural medicine only gradually declined in popularity after the Scientific Revolution (roughly 1543–1700) with its greater privileging of empirical and especially experimental knowledge about the natural world. It persisted in orthodox practice until the mid-nineteenth century, and informed lay explanatory systems into the present. Thus, even the contemporary supremacy of bio-medical orthodoxy is contingent, contested in no small part by medical approaches derived from China and the subcontinent, and by the persistence of holistic European alternatives.

Holism, Humouralism, and Globalism: From Orthodoxy to Heterodoxy

The broad similarities between medical thought in East Asia, the Indian subcontinent, and Europe endured into the eighteenth century, despite the quite culturally specific models of the body-microcosm postulated by each system. All three systems—and any secular but unsystematized competitors—depended for their explanatory and interpretative power on substances, structures, and analogies demanded by overarching theoretical models; their sources of evidence too were drawn from essentially the same points of access to the body and its functions. In this way, medicine in the pre-modern world challenges what we see as entrenched distinctions between 'alternative' and 'orthodox', and between 'western' and 'non-western' medicine. These distinctions depend on the existence (and wide acceptance) of strict boundaries between the different categories of medical practice. But humoural medicine, wherever practised, was a broad church: it could include insights from many quarters, and idiosyncrasy in all. Healers across the medical spectrum in each of the major systems I've examined might offer the same patient a different diagnosis and therapy, but all used similar systems of explanation to justify their prescriptions. Thus, language barriers notwithstanding, doctors from around the globe could appreciate the medical thinking of their distant peers, and in many cases could draw upon it.

Sir John Floyer, for example, writing in England in 1701, drew heavily upon Chinese pulse diagnosis and prognosis to support his arguments in favour of a 'physician's pulse watch'. In his treatise, he explicitly compared and contrasted the European and Chinese arts of reading the pulse:

In the general description of China by the Embassy from the Dutch East India Company, I find this account 'as to Physick and Chyrurgery they are Experts, and their rules of the Art differ not much from those of the European Physicians; for at first they feel the pulse like them, and are skillful in discovering by the same the inward distempers of the body . . .'[15]

Floyer tried explain and synthesize the Chinese and western accounts of the pulse and the body. Crucially, he began this task with the presumption that each was describing the same human body, and that practitioners of each system were equally rational. When he came across apparent contradictions between the systems—or when the translated Chinese text he was reading seemed to him nonsensical—he glossed the Chinese in accordance with western assumptions about the body. Of course, this process was not without its problems. Floyer often discarded or rewrote Chinese theories which were not consistent with European, anatomically informed, ideas of the body.

'Tis ridiculous to believe that the pulse can depend in its alterations on the solid parts of any viscera, but it does evidently alter by the fluids; therefore, 'tis obvious that the Chinese respect the fluids, which are secreted by those parts in feeling of the pulse; and if this be a fair conjecture, I have probably accommodated the Chinese and Grecian art of feeling the pulse.[16]

Though he clearly privileged anatomy and its evidence, Floyer did not accept his contemporaries' claims for the supremacy of the anatomical approach to the body unquestioningly. He noted rather astringently that,

Tho' neither the *Greeks* nor the *Chinese* knew the true Fabrick of the Organs of the Pulse, nor their true action and uses, nor the circulation of humours, and the causes of it, yet the *Greeks* discovered the polses of all diseases and humours, and passions: And the *Chinese* their Art of Physic [based] on the pulse and its differences . . . [17]

Floyer concluded, in essence, that a pulse by any name (or studied through any interpretive system) would beat as revealing a rhythm of sickness or health:

I would plainly ask whether the art of the pulse be not the same whether we call the causes by the Chinese, Grecian, or Modern names? The different names or hypothesis are fram'd and built after divers experiments have been try'd, and matters of fact clearly observ'd; and the hypothesis is always well adapted to the natural phenomena, and we may practice the Chinese as well as the old Grecian notions . . . [18]

In other words, since all of these doctrines of the pulse were based on the same 'matters of fact', they were necessarily compatible and complementary. And as I've argued, they did share significant insights and intellectual approaches, at least up to the period in which John Floyer wrote. But even as the expansion of global trading networks and the emergence of new empires greatly increased contact between medical systems (through eroding the geographical barriers between cultures), changes in European medicine during the long eighteenth century also raised and reinforced boundary walls between European and non-European medical practices, beliefs, and practitioners. The slow, contingent, and highly contested construction of a new orthodoxy in medicine had begun: the new medicine would be rooted in notions of 'science' and experiment, rather than scholarship and experience, and it would displace to the periphery much of the previously shared substance of global medical systems. With it, the era of free and *equal* medical exchange between the Europe and the rest of the world was coming to an end (at least temporarily). The 'Jesuit bark'—the bark of the South American cinchona tree—offers a fine example of the new medical globalism which was emerging in its place, one in which there was much more rapid exchange and interchange between medical systems and cultures, but also much more rigid intellectual boundaries between them.

Cinchona bark (now known to be a rich source of the anti-malarial drug quinine) was brought back to Europe in the first half of the seventeenth century. It was a powerful therapy against the fevers that rendered the tropical world so dangerous for Europeans; knowledge of its medical utility was, of course, derived from indigenous medical knowledge. As the product of a tropical plant, the bark reinforced the older providential belief in a merciful divinity who had ensured that the diseases of a region could be cured by that region's own natural productions. This belief, as well as more mundane factors—for example, the presence of both diseases and materia medica unfamiliar to the western medical tradition—had long encouraged Europeans abroad to observe indigenous healing practices actively and attentively, and to adopt them on a more or less equal footing with western practices. Thus, the bark was exported at great volume and sold for substantial profits in Europe as a general febrifuge (though quinine is only effective against malaria), and entered into the standard medical repertoire at home and abroad. As the eighteenth century progressed, however, European mercantilism—with its emphasis on creating (or commandeering) markets that could be controlled by a single nation-state—deepened into the beginnings of imperialism. In this climate, while local medical knowledge remained an important resource in practice, medicine as a representative aspect of culture (with technology and science) became, in Adas's memorable phrase, 'the measure of men'. Europeans suffered no doubts as to which 'men'—which civilization—came out at the top of the measuring scale: European models of natural knowledge and medicine were the standard by which all cultures would be measured. Under this new rubric, Europeans continued to observe non-western medical systems closely. However, the observer's gaze was no longer primarily acquisitive but instead critical, assessing, and increasingly jaundiced. Thus, over the course of the long eighteenth century, non-European medical practices were studied first as a providential resource (and one necessary to enable national agendas of settlement and trade); then a source of potential commodities and profit; and finally as a metric for assessing the relative standing and progress of civilizations. The changing significance of non-western medical expertise over the course of the century was reflected in the types of observations made, how they were presented, and the responses they elicited in Europe itself.

For all Swift's scoffing, the eighteenth century saw the emergence of a range of newly demonstrable, but nonetheless invisible natural forces or substances: dephlogisticated air/phlogiston (oxygen), magnetism, galvanism (or electricity), and mesmerism (each of these latter three forces were regarded as the effect of some as yet unidentified fluid). In medicine, these substances could be easily integrated with the humoural tradition as 'imponderable' or 'subtle' fluids (analogous to substances like *ojas* or *qi,* and the classical *pneuma*). As such, they would naturally have strong and direct impacts on the body and bodily health, and therefore come within the purview of medicine. And indeed, among the earliest experiments with each imponderable were those relating to potential or proposed medical uses.

However, newer models of the body also addressed themselves to the new subtle fluids, and were strengthened by them. These models drew upon the Baconian experimentalist tradition, Renaissance interest in anatomical dissection, and the rising tides of mechanism (the *philosophe*-physician Julien La Mettrie, for instance, described the body as 'a machine that winds its own springs'[19]) and materialism. The hydraulic model of the body, rooted in Harvey's celebrated discovery of the circulation of the blood, persisted in popularity. Alternatively, physicians could focus on the nervous system (the structures and functions of which were undergoing rapid elucidation by dissection and comparative anatomy) and its manifest qualities of irritability and sensibility. And mechanism in this era began its battle with vitalism to control understandings of the life force, and/or consciousness. The new fluids became the highly visible tools and spoils of this struggle. Meanwhile rising faith in progress brought with it increasing (albeit rather hypocritical, given western medicine's long-standing preoccupation with Galenism) contempt for apparent stasis, for 'hidebound tradition' in medicine, as elsewhere in the social milieu. This had a highly damaging effect on western perceptions of non-western medical systems with their continued regard for tradition and established scholarly knowledge.

As ever, changing attitudes towards the production of knowledge and facts in medicine only slowly altered medical practice. To the frustration of medical practitioners and consumers alike, the new knowledge of the body offered by anatomy, physiology, and the like could only rarely be turned to therapeutic ends. This is not to say that the eighteenth century was a time of therapeutic stasis; new treatments did emerge, ranging from Jenner's technique of vaccination to widespread experimentation with medical electricity. Surgical outcomes improved as dissection became gradually a more common feature of medical training: surgeons more familiar with the body's interior operated faster, more efficiently, and with less blood loss. Globally, Europeans were gathering, propagating, and exchanging medical products and information with more cultures and in greater detail than ever before, albeit with a newly hierarchical and extractive zeal. Meanwhile, the medical market-place at home was both buoyant and resilient, incorporating new medical ideas and products without discarding the old. Like Newton's physics, the new modes of medicine—in particular, the emergence of the 'clinic' and of physical examination as an adjunct to the (still far more important) interrogative patient history—were regarded by many as faddish (and in Britain, as dangerously Frenchified, reductionist, and threatening to the doc-tor–patient relationship). Indeed, from the perspective of the late eighteenth and early nineteenth century, the medical system we have embraced—with its stress on exclusive knowledge and ma-terialist interpretations of disease, its marked specializations and emphasis on cure (as opposed to either prevention or care)—was neither more nor less than one medical sect within the broad category of 'regular' medicine.

The presumption that medicine could or should be, above all, 'scientific' in fact dates to the late nineteenth century—and achieved the status of orthodoxy more recently still, perhaps only in the inter-war period. Experience as the most reliable source of natural know-ledge was only gradually displaced by 'experiment'. And the notion that medical knowledge—knowledge about the body, behaviour, health, and disease—should properly be universal, absolute, and 'objective', rather than individual, contingent, and 'subjective' was laboriously produced, by medical elites, public health officials, social reformers, imperialists, and others, over the course of the entire nineteenth and early twentieth century. The remaining chapters of this volume will examine in detail the emergence of both alternative and orthodox medical systems, and the role played by each in the integration or rejection of global medical expertise. At present, it is therefore necessary only to note a few of the more important characteristics and trends of nineteenth-century medicine.

If the eighteenth century presents a vision of medicine as a commodity of the marketplace, and embodiment (in health or sickness) as a franchise shared between practitioners and patients, the nineteenth exhibits medicine as one, or perhaps more accurately, as several, professions, all competing for exclusive rights to interpret and prescribe bodily experience. The theoretical fluidity and syncretism of Enlightenment medicine gave way to a medical culture marked by competing sects, each with its own overarching theory, and each claiming a monopoly on true knowledge of the body and disease. It was this combination of system-building (an outgrowth largely of Enlightenment commitments to a rational and reasoned medicine) and increasing rigidity—a sort of medical monotheism—that initially produced the division we now take for granted between 'alternative' and 'orthodox' medicine. In this contentious atmosphere, the epithet of 'quack' was reserved no longer for those who practised medicine solely for lucre but was freely applied by the proponents of any one system to the proponents of all others. The essential problem, as I will illustrate in subsequent chapters, was that the theories of the body on which medical systems like homeopathy, allopathy, chiropractic, and osteopathy were based were mutually exclusive. One could not readily abide by the rule that like cured like and yet accept the argument that all diseases stemmed from disorders of the skeletal system. Still less could followers of homeopathy or osteopathy accommodate the long-established belief that one should treat a symptom or disease with its opposite.

In laying claim to the status of profession, practitioners of medicine whatever their system also sought to assert their authority over the body (in all aspects of life). In doing so, they began to displace the patient's experience of his or her illness from the foreground of diagnosis and prognosis. This experiential, subjective account of illness was replaced with an account based instead on the practitioner's observations—gained increasingly through physical and technologically mediated examination of the patient's body—and exclusive knowledge. That knowledge was no longer rooted primarily in theory and scholarship, but in the highly material world of the charnel house, the hospital, and by the end of the century, the laboratory. From these institutions, supercharged by competition and monopolistic ambition within the medical world and by the exigencies of urbanization, empire, and the consequent rise of state interest in matters of health, would flow the major innovations of the century: surgical anaesthesia, germ theory, anti- and then a-sepsis. By the end of the nineteenth century, 'scientific medicine' was ascendant (though not monolithic). Rapid profes- sionalization, though important to the survival of other nineteenth- century medical systems, was not enough to preserve the visibility and status they had achieved; the weight of state intervention in medicine tipped the balance in favour of an orthodox biomedical monopoly. If epidemic and infectious diseases could not yet be cured, they could in theory be prevented by state-sanctioned and -funded public health measures designed to fight the filth and contagion of germs. Despite continuing pressure from 'alternative' medicine, and from conservatives within orthodox medicine itself, by the end of the nineteenth century, the new 'scientific' medicine was perceived by a growing number of doctors and patients alike as both authoritative and powerful.

The twentieth century saw what might be called the industrial- ization of medicine. It was marked by rapid increases in the complexity of medical organization and technologies, and in the number of specializations—already burgeoning by the end of the nineteenth century. Hospitals, still in the late nineteenth century regarded by many as places of last resort in medical care (and thus serving mainly the poor), became the central institution of medical practice and education, and prominent research sites. But medical research found a home too in industry, in universities, and in governmental organizations of various types, ranging from public health labora- tories to military installations. The twentieth century also witnessed the rise of third-party payers and, particularly in Western Europe, national health services. In either case, a new entity obtruded itself into the doctor–patient relationship. Moreover, in the wake of the bacteriological revolution of the late nineteenth and early twentieth century and the decline of infectious disease, chronic and degenerative diseases—conditions characterized by long-term morbidity and often pain, rather than acute disease and sudden death—emerged as the major objects of medical interventions. And it is in relation to precisely these conditions that alternative medicine has returned to the forefront of medical culture. Ironically, biomedicine's initial victory over infectious disease cast into sharp relief its inability to cure the chronically ill and ageing. At the same time, the rigours of biomedicine from the patients' perspective—the degree to which it was impersonal, driven by and constructed around the needs of the laboratory and technology (not to mention the interests of what some commentators have called the medical-industrial complex), and disease- rather than patient-focused—provoked many to accuse both the medical system and its practitioners of arrogance, insensitivity, and greed.

Orthodoxy in medicine—as in all fields of endeavour—must be built and continually rebuilt in response to changes in environment, knowledge, social mores, and cultural assumptions. The process of creating such a consensus is complicated for medicine by a series of paradoxes. Medical knowledge addresses natural, physical phenomena—'the real world'. And today, laypersons and professionals alike commonly regard medical knowledge as 'objective'—dispassionate, unbiased, and free of unacknowledged assumptions. Yet medical knowledge is also deeply inscribed by culture, precisely because its 'natural' subjects, the human body, health, and disease are foci of intense cultural scrutiny and control. Consider for example, the case of the physical examination. Today, medical professionals—and medical professionals alone—have the unquestioned right to examine our bodies by touching and by direct observation. Orthodox medical practice depends heavily on this level of access to the patient's body: the very notion of 'objective' diagnosis (crucial to the authority of orthodox medicine) is based on direct physician (and technician/machine) observation and measurement, rather than patient self-reporting. Obviously cultural attitudes towards the body can constrain this form of contact, particularly between men and women. But cultural attitudes towards the medical profession too can affect the medical prerogative of touch: if orthodox professionals lose the trust of the public for whatever reason, then their exemption from cultural rules governing physical contact too will be under scrutiny. Conversely, as alternative therapists professionalize and gain in public status and trust, they are increasingly granted the licence over the body that has been for almost a century the exclusive right of the medically qualified.

The loud and largely consistent authority claims, and distinctive styles of knowledge production and practice displayed by contemporary orthodox medicine also renders its differences with other therapeutic systems and practices highly visible. Because biomedicine positions itself as possessing absolute knowledge—knowledge that is true for and of all bodies, everywhere, independent of culture—its proponents tend to resist claims to parity made by other medical systems. Practitioners who hold different medical beliefs, or who practise medicine, or produce medical knowledge in other ways must therefore generally choose between positioning themselves and their medical practices as either 'complementary' or 'alternative' to biomedicine. Each position entails accepting a certain relationship to medical orthodoxy. If practitioners choose to regard their practices as 'complementary' to biomedicine, then they are accepting a more or less subordinate place within the orthodox hierarchy. The 'complementary' label accepts the universalizing claims of biomedicine; this has obvious implications in turn for the truth status of the 'complementary' system (particularly if it rests on another culture's cosmology and body model). On the other hand, the label 'alternative' expresses an oppositional relationship between the system or practice to which it is applied, and biomedicine. Although this category resists incorporation and assimilation with biomedicine, and therefore escapes a lower status in the biomedical hierarchy of knowledge, it also hinders acceptance into the institutions of medical orthodoxy—the loci of most medical care in contemporary society.

So where do the medical systems of other cultures fit onto this spectrum? Until the late eighteenth century, all medicine was largely subjective—rooted in the patient's experience of his or her illness, and

in the healer's experience recognizing and treating similar constellations of symptoms and circumstance. With the 'rise of science' and the
professionalization of orthodox medicine came a rejection of purely
experiential and empirical knowledge. This rejection began with the
exclusion of the patient's experience of disease, the diminution of the
patient's authority over his or her own bodily knowledge. It eventually
extended even to the experience of physicians. The West did not
attempt to develop a science of the subjective, of the experiential. But
this was an artefact of culture, perhaps a reflection of western distaste
for the embodied, sensational world, and of western privileging of the
gaze alone. Certainly, other cultures did not choose to forgo the
powerful tools of subjective perception of the body in their medicine
or evaluations of the natural world: consider *qigong*, meditation, and
other therapeutic practices dependent on the embodied mind. And as
these cultures came to the attention of the West, so too did their
medical systems. For example, from the late seventeenth to the late
nineteenth century, westerners began to explore traditional (but even
today scientifically inexplicable) Chinese techniques like moxabustion
and acupuncture (see Chapters 1 and 3). This was exactly the period
in which western medicine began to marginalize subjective experience—particularly patients' experiences of their own bodies—as a kind
of authoritative knowledge about the natural world. As this process of
downgrading the subjective gathered pace in western medical thought
and education, the value of purely empirical knowledge too came
under question: if you could not explain why a medical phenomenon
occurred, its value as evidence was ever-diminished—at least in theory. In medical practice, of course, both the subjective and the empirical remained, and remain, pretty hard to ignore.

But not all western medical systems gave up on embodied
knowledge as a source of medical and curative insight. Two of
the most popular western medical innovations of the late eighteenth
and nineteenth centuries depended heavily on subjective experience
as a source of data and of proof. Homeopathy placed considerable
trust in the experiential: its hallmark doctrine of *similia similibus
curantur* ('like treats like'), for example, relied on homeopathic
physicians accurately reporting their self-induced symptoms after

experimentally consuming a potential drug (see Chapter 2). And mesmerism, or animal magnetism, occupied a fascinating middle ground between exclusive reliance on 'objective' and external readings of the body, and 'subjective' and internal ones (see Chapters 2 and 4). In mesmerism, the hypnotized patients themselves became the experimental instruments. Their self-reports while under the mesmeric influence were taken by the therapy's medical and lay supporters as 'objective' data not merely about the hypnotic state but about the conditions for which they were being treated. Even today, the role of subjective states like optimism and 'will to live' are well recognized within biomedicine as important predictors of patient survival rates in serious illness and trauma.

So: medical policy-makers, practitioners, and consumers alike are faced with the extravagant costs and proliferating bureaucracies of 'objective' biomedicine in the twenty-first century; with increasing public suspicion and even resentment of the authoritative stance and impersonal mien encouraged by a century of biomedical near-monopoly; and with burgeoning popular interest in the more holistic and experiential medicine of other cultures. What impact has this winter of discontent already had on the cultures of medicine in the West, and what effects may reasonably be predicted?

In the account with which this chapter opened, a layman was able to present in the medical press his own evidence and arguments supporting the adoption by orthodox medicine of an originally heterodox—in fact cross-cultural—therapy. In succeeding chapters, I will sketch out the historical processes by which practitioners and patients (among others) crafted western responses to alternative medicines from a range of cultures. Today, patients and the lay public are much less empowered to intervene in the practice of medicine than they were at the beginning of the nineteenth century. However, if patients are less able to sponsor innovations in orthodox medicine, they remain powerful advocates for alternative, complementary, and cross-cultural medicine. This in turn is a potent force in the modern medical marketplace, a marketplace every bit as vibrant, competitive, lucrative, and baroque in its institutions and tastes as that of the eighteenth century.

'WHAT IS THIS BURNING?'

In 1662 at the Dutch settlement in Batavia (now Jakarta, Indonesia), the minister Hermann Busschof took to his bed: 'I laboured under an extraordinary pain in both my knees and feet, not knowing whither to turn my self for pain, having used in vain all those means by which I had formerly found some ease.'[1] Busschof's extended attack drove him to desperate measures. After six weeks of agony and sleeplessness, Busschof was persuaded 'to suffer an Indian Doctress to come to me, (whom my wife commonly employed for the curing of our slaves . . .)'. This 'Doctress' immediately recognized Busschof's illness and claimed that she could easily cure it. Busschof was delighted—until she told him the method she used. Although a fixture of orthodox medicine in Asia, her technique—subsequently called moxabustion in the West—clearly sounded harsh to European ears: 'to tell you the truth, it was done by a way of Burning: which means being by me rejected out of an apprehension I had of the pain that must needs to accompany such a remedy. . . . I could not then resolve upon it'. Horrified, Busschof sent the healer away; her treatment might be good enough for native slaves, who were anyway hardened to it, but it was unsuitable for more civilized and sensitive European bodies.

Busschof was once again alone with the travails of his disease. He began to regret his timidity almost as soon as the healer had left his bedside. He described himself as desperate, 'longing' to see her again, and on her return, he steeled himself for her caustic fire.

I would suffer her to try her art and skill on me; which having at last agreed unto, she went presently to work; having demanded a lighted candle, and solicitously search'd for that part of the place affected where the greatest pain

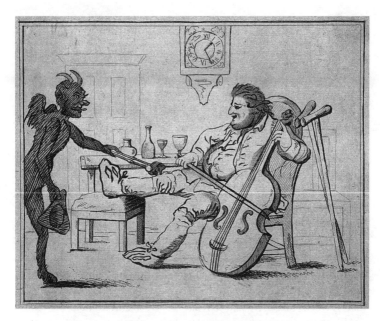

9. 'The Origin of the Gout', Henry William Bunbury, 1785. Bunbury's drawing perfectly illustrates contemporary understandings of the cause of gout—drink, self-indulgence, and excesses of the table—and its typical victim: prosperous men of middle years. The devil burning his knee represents both the fiery pain of the ailment and its association with sins of the flesh.

was: and thereupon she burned with her Moxa . . . on my feet and knees . . . without raising any blisters, or causing any after-pain; whereupon all the pain . . . vanish'd. All this operation was finish'd in less than half an hour, without any bodies hearing me complain of pain. And I herewith declare, that even whilst the burning lasted, I found myself much inclined to sleep . . .

Busschof was afflicted with the immobilizing, agonizing, and yet (even then) faintly comic disease, gout. This was a particularly unfortunate diagnosis for a Protestant minister, since gout was a disease strongly associated with excesses of the table, the bottle, and the bedchamber (see Figure 9). Busschof's ready access to non-western medicine was unusual, but the situation which provoked his choice was not: 'regular' western medicine had failed to cure him of an incapacitating illness, and in desperation he cast around for other options, in this case, the 'regular' medicine of a different culture. Its success gave Busschof much to consider—and much to question—in western medicine: 'and first of all [called] into question, whether physicians hitherto have had a right notion, and given a true account of the nature and qualities of this disease'.

So let's take another look at Asian medicine, this time through the eyes of Hermann Busschof and his contemporaries, Europeans engaging either directly or indirectly with the non-European world and non-European medicine in the long eighteenth century. In many ways, they are not very different from us. Like us, eighteenth-century Europeans lived in a world that was rapidly becoming smaller as new technologies, new enterprises, and new political exigencies rendered it more accessible. They witnessed a constant stream of new and exotic medicines and therapies entering the marketplace. Western innovators and entrepreneurs produced some of these novelties; others emerged from the non-western cultures with which Europeans were increasingly in contact. Like contemporary westerners, our eighteenth-century counterparts combined great faith in their own culture's medical cosmology and techniques with a healthy scepticism of doctors' claims to treat specific cases or illnesses successfully. The latter attitude made Enlightenment Europeans willing, even eager, to experiment with novel practices; the former inclined them to interpret those practices in the light of existing western model of the body, health, and disease.

Our focus will be on two therapies whose long histories in Europe may seem surprising: moxabustion and acupuncture. Both techniques depend on a model of the body very different from those prevailing in Europe in the seventeenth and eighteenth centuries, and even more different from the biomedical model we rely upon today. This is one factor that makes their early transmission (and indeed their contemporary popularity) seem unlikely: medical practices are typically culturally specific—that is, they are intellectually coherent with and practically responsive to the cultures in which they initially developed. Look, for example, at the increasing medical emphasis on anatomical knowledge in eighteenth-century

Western Europe. The incorporation of dissection into medical training and knowledge production was closely integrated with Enlightenment ideals of rationalism and empiricism. But the Enlightenment was also characterized by calls for greater equality between individuals and groups, and for an end to bigotry rooted in custom and religion. In practice, Enlightenment ideals mandated the political, social, and economic enfranchisement of all rational beings—potentially including women, the lower classes, and ethnic and religious minorities. Anatomy offered elites a way around these logical, but socially disruptive, conclusions. By painting a picture of immutable 'natural' difference between the sexes, races, and eventually classes, anatomy offered an acceptable rationale for excluding women, non-whites, and other groups from the franchise. The social utility of this medical knowledge in turn allowed anatomy-based styles of medicine to gain still greater social authority.

This kind of seamless fit with their native cultures often causes medical systems and practices to mesh poorly with other cultures. For example, anatomy, if it is to be useful in the production of medical knowledge, demands copious human dissection. It was therefore wildly unsuited to cultures like that of China (in which ancestor-worship and Confucian law rendered the bodies of the dead sacrosanct) or India, where contact with the dead was for many ritually polluting. But the great authority given to anatomical knowledge and models of the body in the West (even before such knowledge had produced clinical benefits) made the western profession highly sceptical of the alternative visions of the body put forward by non-anatomizing cultures. Thus Indian and Chinese reluctance to dissect human bodies became a substantial barrier to the acceptance of either Indian or Chinese medical theories by western doctors (though it did not necessarily bar the acceptance of Indian or Chinese medical practices and pharmacopoeia).

Acupuncture and moxabustion in seventeenth- and eighteenth-century China (and in the 'Traditional Chinese Medicine' practised in Europe and North America today) were therapies predicated on a set of basic philosophical beliefs about the natural world (see Introduction). Chinese scholar-physicians used this cosmology to interpret their broad empirical knowledge of the human body and disease, and from this combination of experience and interpretation produced an immense pharmacopoeia, a detailed disease classification system, and a set of body-maps. These maps, central to the practice of both techniques, define relationships between the body's surface and organ systems, mediated through a circulatory system that moves both tangible and intangible substances (and in particular the vital energy, *qi*) around the body. At certain points on the body's surface, the various vessels or channels through which these fluids move, and which connect different functional and sensory organs, can be stimulated, thereby altering the flows of *qi* within them and between the organs. In moxabustion, this is done through the medium of small cones of fibre (extracted from the leaves of *Artemesia vulgaris* or mugwort) that are burnt on top of the points. In acupuncture, needles, inserted to different depths and sometimes manipulated, are the means of intervention.

European medicine itself was neither monolithic nor hegemonic before the later nineteenth century (see Chapter 3). Patients, practitioners, and quacks did all share a basic understanding of the body—the humoural model discussed in the Introduction—and were increasingly aware of the explanatory potential of human anatomy. But this shared model was very flexible; understandings of the nature of the humours, their actions in causing or mediating disease, and their relationships with both the environment and different medical interventions were subject to interpretation and reinterpretation by all parties in the medical encounter. Moreover, although Europeans (particularly among Europe's elites) did look to trained/experienced physicians and surgeons for treatment, those groups had no monopoly on healing, and indeed provided a minority of medical care. Europe's patients actively sought new therapeutic choices—medicine was increasingly like any other consumer good in the 'age of consumption'. Furthermore, the commercial, as well as the therapeutic, success of the 'Jesuit bark' (quinine-rich cinchona, see Introduction) provided European travellers and traders with all the evidence they needed that a new remedy could be readily converted into profit. Thus much of the medical information gathered by westerners abroad addressed herbal medicines, and drew on the novel (to Europeans) pharmacopoeia of the tropics. However, as Busschof's encounter with the local Doctress suggests, other forms of medical expertise were also tapped by desperate (or simply curious) European voyagers. In an age when European medicine was regularly the butt of satirical humour for its painful and poisonous inefficacy, these exotic cures were well worth writing home about, and provided considerable matter for discussion and debate among physicians, philosophers, and lay elites alike.

'The Effect Will Soon Silence You': (Re)Discovering Moxabustion

Busschof joined this multilayered—for it pervaded popular, medical, and scholarly sources in this period—debate enthusiastically. He presented the conclusions he had drawn from his encounter with another culture's medicine as a lively question and answer session between himself and a doubtful reader. The volume was popular enough to appear in multiple editions and several translations, including an English version, published in 1676.[2] In the book, Busschof's imaginary interlocutor stood in for European patients and professionals alike, and expressed the doubts that Busschof predicted and hoped to calm in his European audience. Thus it is a powerful lens through which to inspect popular eighteenth-century attitudes towards the medicine of other cultures, and to explore the degree to which they resemble or differ from our own.

Busschof anticipated considerable scepticism about a cure originating so far from home. He argued that the success of therapeutic burning could and should teach the western profession about the nature of gout, and chastised European doctors for their arrogance in disregarding the expertise of other cultures. He even hinted that religious bigotry might underpin dismissive European attitudes:

[Q.] But pray tell me, Sir, what's the reason that this burning hath been so many years hid from us Europeans, whereas it hath been experienced for so vast a time in those Indian kingdoms, where it is so common . . . ? A. This is to be imputed to the carelessness and conceitedness of the Europeans, because having so good an opinion of themselves, they are ashamed to learn any good thing from those Pagans; as if they alone were possessed of all knowledge, and those nations had no share at all in it.[3]

The efficacy of moxa certainly contradicted the models of gout offered by western medicine, and Busschof presented as preferable his own interpretation of Chinese understandings of the disease. He knew his audience well enough to guess what its next objections would be: 'But when the physitians [sic] of Europe and other parts from hence have better understood the nature of the Gout, will they not be able to find out a better remedy against it?' Busschof was adamant: '[T]hey will never find out any better remedy than this burning with Moxa . . .'.

Busschof expected more pragmatic objections as well. In the seventeenth century, as today, ensuring patient compliance with medical regimen was a matter of grave professional concern. Elite (and opinion-shaping) patients had considerable control over the doctor–patient encounter, based both on the power of the purse and on the fact that much knowledge of the body and disease was held in common by professionals and laity alike. Such patients could not be commanded, but could only be persuaded to accept both the sinified model of gout, and the moxabustion treatment itself. Busschof argued that careful explanation of the technique and the new understanding of gout could even overcome the reluctance of patients who had already experienced 'that kind of burning which hither to hath been used in Europe [which] hath made men very averse from that way'.[4]

In presenting the West with a therapy drawn from a separate and very different medical culture, Busschof also had to fight against the importance of historical—and particularly classical—pedigree as a source of authority in medicine. Within the medical elites of the day, a violent debate was already brewing over the relative merits of classical and contemporary medical knowledge. However, from the perspective of an educated layman like Busschof, the authority of precedent was still a powerful argument against his innovation, and one which he had to address: '[Q.] But many doctors and Chirurgeons are like to condemn this remedy as new and unknown, and so render it suspected among their patients?' Busschof's alter ego called upon the value of experienced relief to disarm this straw-man: 'The effect will soon silence you, and convince you of envy and ignorance [on the part of the protesting medical men].'

Busschof accompanied his sharp critique of western medicine's 'arrogance' and resistance to change with some censure of medicine in Asia. Like many of the scientific and medical observers who followed him, Busschof regarded East Asian medicine as fatally flawed by a superstitious regard for tradition:

[Q.] Do these nations cure themselves and others of the Gout, surely and speedily? A. No they do not, except it be casually . . . Q. What's the matter, seeing that they have possessed this excellent means of burning from immemorial times? A. 'Tis not the want of a good remedy, but their stubbornness, superstition, and perverse custom, that they do not cure the gout but by chance or good fortune. For they have been taught indeed to burn in very many, and yet in certain determined and prescribed places of the body; not being to be induced to transgress those prescriptions, though the pain should require it.[5]

Of course this criticism, though framed in terms of East Asian medicine, equally sternly rebuked those westerners who rejected new or empirically successful treatments solely because they were not authorized by classical precedent, or came from non-Christian culture! And it is no coincidence that Busschof's enthusiasm for moxabustion sprang from its efficacy in treating the gout, nor that his disaffection for western practices crystallized around its particu-lar failings in relation to that condition. Gout struck the middle and upper classes at mid-life; it was painful and incapacitating, but rarely fatal; its precise nature and definition had been noisily debated since classical times; and there was no accepted consensus on its causes or mode of action. In each of these attributes—and in its prominence in contemporary medical debate—gout typifies diseases that have attracted therapeutic investigation and innovation, whether quack, orthodox, cross-cultural, or self-consciously 'alternative'. Thus the relationship between gout, gout-sufferers, gout-doctors, and the practice of medicine illustrates wider patterns of medical system-building.

Today in the West, alternative, complementary, and cross-cultural medicines have come to prominence in the treatment of conditions which are common, highly visible, chronic, generally not life-threatening, and intractable to the usual techniques of biomedicine. For example, acupuncture is applied for lower back pain, homeopathists treat asthma and allergies, hypnotism is popular with those fighting addiction to nicotine, and herbal medicines address depression. Like these conditions, gout was an important disease in the late seventeenth and eighteenth centuries, for both commercial and intellectual reasons. It also clearly demonstrates the relationship between medical failure, disease intractability, and the transmission of medical knowledge across cultural boundaries. Physicians in the seventeenth and eighteenth centuries disagreed violently (with all comers) about how—or indeed whether—to treat gout. For example, Thomas Sydenham (1624–89), 'the English Hippocrates', expressed grave reservations about many of the long-established therapies used to avert or dispel the gout in 'regular' medicine. He worried that potent drugs would only cause the dangerous gouty matter to move from its safe, if painful, lodging in the joints to the blood and hence to the viscera, 'and so endangers the life of the patient, who was quite safe before'.[6] As his theory suggests, many 'regular' physicians regarded gout as a salutary sickness, one that prevented far more serious diseases: 'a fit of the gout terminates symptoms which threaten something worse'.[7]

Because of its perceived prophylactic effects on the body as a whole, many physicians regarded treatment of gout's specific and local symptoms as dangerous to the patient's overall health—and thus as quackish. Indeed, patients were often congratulated by their friends and medical attendants on the occasion of their first attack, as gout was associated with both good breeding and long life. But from the patient's point of view, gout's advantages were gained at substantial cost in time, convenience, and quality of life. Still worse, few of the accepted analgesics were suitable for middle-aged or active sufferers: purging as advised by Hippocrates was dangerous for those no longer youthful; poultices helped the pain, but were regarded as drawing down the humours, and thus weakening the affected joint; plasters dispersed the dangerous and painful humours, but might allow them to move elsewhere in the body, risking other illnesses; rest, warmth, and warm baths carried the same risks—and were hardly ideal choices for the busy man of state; bleeding and sweating were preventives, not cures. Sir William Temple, a prominent English diplomat and gout sufferer, forthrightly dismissed the options available to him in 1677: '[F]or the common Remedies of the Gout, I found exceptions to them all.'[8] Meanwhile sufferers and healers alike despaired of any safe and successful cure: 'it cannot reasonably be assumed that the cure can be accomplished by means of some slight and momentaneous change made in the blood and juices by any kind of medicine or regiment, but the whole constitution is to be altered and the body to be in a manner framed anew'.[9] Indeed, as a chronic disease of the constitution, most regular physicians categorically denied even the possibility of finding a specifically curative medicine for gout: 'As for a cure—this lies, like Truth, *at the bottom of a well*.'[10]

Many medical practitioners shared their clients' dissatisfaction with medicine mired in precedent and authority, and their interest in alternative ways of learning about the natural world. Yet scholastic medicine was backed by classical authority and had relatively high cultural status; it also underpinned patients' expectations about how they would be treated for any given constellation of symptoms, like gout. Physicians had much to lose by lightly dismissing or dangerously deviating from scholarly medical precedent. One book on gout opened with a frank acknowledgement of the bookish conventionality of 'regular' medical practice:

As for my own part, I declare I never more rejoyce, than when I see my patients expectations answer'd, as well as my own: A young practitioner is obliged to keep to the common way, or such as he hath seen practiced, be the effect what it will; I must confess in my younger years, I thought it sufficient to make myself master of the common methods, as practiced by the best modern Authors, I could meet with, and pursued them exactly, with as tolerable success as other practitioners did. . . .[11]

It is therefore unsurprising that much interest in alternative forms of medicine came from surgeons, and 'irregulars'. They had less to lose, and much to gain—particularly if the innovations they proposed or adopted from other cultures opened up new commercial territories. As a systemic disease, gout was properly treated by regimen (a planned way of life designed to improve health, and usually incorporating regulated diets, exercise, and actual medicines)—the therapeutic province of physicians. But if an external and local remedy like moxabustion could effectively cure so complex a disease, then surgeons—who, after all, specialized in external and local treatments—could rightly claim a commercial and intellectual stake in one of the most important and paradigmatic diseases of their day. Neither group had much success in creating an effective or accepted therapy. However, their attention and efforts may have had an effect on patient attitudes towards the disease and its cure, by rendering more visible the degree of medical uncertainty and debate that surrounded gout.

Temple claimed to have seen a great and widespread increase in gout during his lifetime. He argued that this trend was made particularly dangerous by gout's unusual demographics: it spared women, the poor, and the young to attack wealthy men at the height of their powers. Gout seemed to seek out the most powerful men of government affairs and the military, disturbing their minds as well as their comfort. As Temple noted, these men were rarely under 40, 'at about which time, the natural heat beginning to decay, makes room for those distempers they are most inclined to by their Native Constitutions, or by their customs and habits of life'.[12] And those constitutions, in Temple's experience, were likely to be weakened either by the luxurious taint of high birth, or by the excessive indulgences common to those newly enjoying the perquisites of power. In choosing men to fill powerful roles, therefore, Temple urged the State 'to consider their bodies as well as their minds, and ages and health as well as their abilities ... [P]ublic business comes to suffer by private infirmities ... I have seen ... the pulse of the Government beat high or low with that of the Governour.'[13] No man, he argued, could reach the age of 50, 'without feeling his journey in all parts, whatever distinctions are made between the mind and the body, or between judgment and memory'.[14]

Temple's own experience of gout confirmed him in these opinions. He first fell ill just as he was about to travel on urgent diplomatic business. Urgency and, as Temple put it, 'obstinacy' and 'sullenness' with Europe's elite scholastic medicine drove him, albeit unwillingly, to try a new remedy which had come his way. 'I never thought it would have befallen me to be the first that should try a new experiment . . . being little inclined to practise upon others, and as little that others should practise upon me.'[15] And experiment he did—but his 'sullenness' extended even to the most unusual wares of the European medical marketplace. Instead Temple was persuaded by a friend to try an exotic technique only recently imported from the East, 'the *Indian* way of Curing the Gout by *Moxa*':[16] Temple's later description of the therapy gives us some idea of how strange and improbable its claims must have seemed to him:

[Moxa] was a certain kind of Moss that grew in the *East-Indies*; . . . their way was, when ever any body fell into a Fit of the Gout, to take a small quantity of it, and form it into a figure, broad at the bottom as a two-pence, and pointed at the top; To set the bottom exactly upon the place where the violence of the pain was fixed, then with a small round perfumed Match . . . to give fire to the top of the Moss; which by burning down by degrees, came at length to the skin, and burnt it till the Moss was consumed to ashes; That many times the first burning would remove the pain; if not, it was to be renewed a second, third, and fourth time, till it went away, and till the person found he could set his foot boldly to the ground and walk.[17]

Despite this rather unprepossessing description of moxabustion, Temple performed the experiment three times. His persistence is surely a commentary on the dismal state of western treatments for gout. And it was rewarded: after his efforts, he was able to walk again 'without any pain or trouble and much to the surprize of those that were about me, as well as to my own'. His initial scepticism—he noted gloomily that the effect of medical treatment 'seldom reaches to the degree that is promised by the prescribers'—was replaced by amazement: 'this went beyond it, having been applied so late, and the prescription [here referring to the claims made for moxa's efficacy] reaching only to the first attaque of the pain, and before the part begins to swell'.[18]

Moxabustion as Temple depicted it, was truly a remarkable therapy for the eighteenth century: not only did the burning moxa relieve the gout; it did so even when the disease was well established. In other words, moxabustion did not simply ameliorate or prevent gout, but actually cured it. 'The talk of this Cure ran about The Hague, and made the conversation in other places'.[19] Indeed, his cure was so astonishing that Temple's eventual publication of his notes on the subject went through at least four editions, and the popular *London Magazine* published a (slightly garbled) version of Temple's case over seventy years later.[20] Other prominent gout sufferers heard about the technique and tried it themselves with equal success, and Temple (his distaste for experiment apparently overcome in the thrill of the moment) cheerfully tried moxabustion on his maid's toothache, burning several moxas over the vein behind that hapless woman's left ear.

But how had news of this rather exotic alternative reached The Hague in the first place, and what had inspired Temple to try it? In fact, Temple's information originated with Hermann Busschof, in an inversion of the missionary's traditional proselytizing role. Although other travellers in South and East Asia also described moxabustion in their memoirs and travelogues, Busschof was among its most prominent proponents, and was widely cited by the medical profession, including the influential Sydenham. The importance and persuasiveness of his account stems from a combination of factors. First, Busschof experienced moxabustion's curative effects himself. As an educated European (and in England, as a Protestant), his account had greater credibility than either translations of native sources, or descriptions of the technique's effect on non-Europeans. Second, Busschof also sent back with his account the necessary materials for performing moxabustion, and detailed instructions on how to properly use them. Those instructions were drawn from his own first-hand knowledge of the practice of moxabustion in Batavia by an experienced healer, rather than from a scholarly text or second-hand report. Third, he attested to his own successful cure of a disease that was notably intransigent to 'regular' western medicine. At the same time, he supplied a compelling alternative interpretation of that disease, which made sense of the exotic import's efficacy. Drawing upon Asian models, he argued that gout was caused by 'a dry and cold ill-natured damp or vapor, which out of the arteries . . . is driven out into the place that is between the bone and the periostium, distending that most sensible membrane'. This vapour, and the 'preternatural', 'deep-lurking' swelling it caused, produced the 'violent and intolerable' pain of gout.[21]

This explanation of gout in turn rendered moxabustion's curative success explicable in humoural terms. Burning moxas were the ideal treatment: the deeply hidden pockets of icy vapour that caused gout's visible symptoms would be reached or released by moxa's deeply penetrating and ventilating warmth. Moreover, Busschof explicitly positioned moxabustion as preferable to the more usual western surgical remedies for gout—sudorifics, cupping, issues, leeches, or common caustics—the latter four would not reach the malignant vapour 'in its hole', and the former would not fully remove it. Asian moxa was also preferable (because more reliable, safer, and less painful) to the more familiar western cauteries, the hot iron, or the Egyptian method of cautery with nitre-soaked cotton. Finally, Busschof also got the timing right: as Temple pointed out, gout was becoming ever more visible in Europe during this period, while European fascination with and respect for China was also increasing.[22] Indeed, by 1701, enthusiasm for the trappings of Chinese culture was so pronounced, that Sir John Floyer, a British physician and proponent of sphygmanometry (pulse measurement), likened it to the Chinese practice. In support of his new form of standardized pulse diagnosis, he argued: 'I suppose my readers will be pleas'd to practice according to the Chinese mode, as well as to adorn their houses with their curious manufactures, and to use their diet of Thea.'[23]

Moxabustion was a foreign—and, as Busschof's hesitations illustrate, not immediately appealing—medical technique. Assimilating it necessitated changing existing (if contested) medical understandings of a prominent disease. So why were consumers like Temple willing to shelve their own culture's medicine and sample moxa instead? Like many of the elite consumers whose needs, expectations, and demands were influential in shaping medical development throughout this period, Temple was unimpressed by the choices offered him by 'regular' medicine, and highly sceptical of the therapeutic claims of western physicians:

I had past Twenty years of my life, and several accidents of danger in my health, without ANY USE OF PHYSICIANS; and from some experiments of my own, as well as much reading and thought upon that subject, had reasoned myself into an opinion, that the use of them and their methods (unless in some sudden and acute disease) was itself a very great venture, and that their greatest practicers practised least upon themselves, or their friends.[24]

In particular he distrusted the scholastic tradition in western medicine: 'I had ever quarreled with their studying art more than nature, and applying themselves to methods, rather than to remedies; whereas the knowledge of the last is all that nine parts in ten of the world have trusted to in all ages.' In other words, Temple's interest, like Busschof's earlier enthusiasm, was sparked not just by the empirical failure of 'regular' practice, but also by intellectual dissatisfaction with its basis in scholarly knowledge rather than practical—and in today's terms, experimental—experience.

Laymen and -women had much to gain from new approaches to healing. Not only were they offered treatments, rather than exhorted to stoicism or encouraged to count their medical blessings, they might benefit more materially as well. The English translation of Hermann Busschof's tract, for example, carried an interesting notice on its endpapers:

Advertisement.
The Remedies that are required to discharge the Gout, are now to be had of Moses Pitt, at the Angel in St. Paul's Churchyard, Bookseller, with a paper to instruct those that are desirous to learn the way of Burning with Moxa, and to shew the manner thereof; in case there be any body that shall think it not clearly enough delivered in this Book.

By the early nineteenth century, moxa's marketability was established, causing one English commentator to remark rather mournfully on the loss of Java: 'And much indeed is it to be regretted that having once all Java in her possession, England should have abandoned the colony before her enterprising governor had secured all the moxa in the island, as a present to his countrymen, infinitely more valuable than the splendid but inefficacious *Rafflesia*.'[25]

Temple's text also reveals an additional factor in his willingness to adopt a medical treatment from another culture. While his account of moxa acknowledges, even celebrates, its exotic strangeness, Temple also lists more familiar precedents for the therapeutic use of fiery heat. These ranged from ancient Egyptian cautery; to marks found on African slaves indicative of the use of hot irons; to accounts of Inca medicine; to his own childhood experiences of cautery for a putrefied wound, scalding for bruises, and heat for chilblains, as well as 'casual applications of fire to the lower parts' for 'frenzies'. He concluded, 'it was only a tenderness to Mankind that made it less in use amongst us'.[26] In other words, although moxabustion looks utterly unfamiliar to westerners in the twenty-first century, for our seventeenth- and eighteenth-century counterparts, it would have looked like an exotic version of a familiar (if unfashionably archaic) domestic healing practice—and one with a classical pedigree of its own.

Following Busschof's essay and Temple's endorsement of moxabustion, the technique entered European medical discourse, and somewhat more slowly, European medical practice. Scholars at Gresham College in London translated Busschof's volume in 1676, only two years after the Dutch original reached Europe. The translation was immediately reviewed in the *Philosophical Transactions* of the Royal Society (perhaps unsurprisingly, as members of Gresham College were among its most active constituents). By 1693, at least six editions in three languages had been printed. Given this level of interest, it is unsurprising that subsequent travellers and observers in the Far East paid close attention to demonstrations of moxabustion whenever they chanced upon them.

In both English and French sources, Sir William Temple's endorsement of the technique continued to be frequently cited through the eighteenth century, usually alongside Busschof and more recent medical accounts. But what effect did their respective experiences of cross-cultural medicine have on Herman Busschof and William Temple? Were there any significant differences between the 'moxabustion' of a European treated by a skilled indigenous practitioner in a country where it was commonplace, and that portrayed by a Sinophile receiving his therapy from a European practitioner who had learned the technique from a book? In other words, do different patterns of exposure to cross-cultural medical expertise provoke or facilitate different responses?

Both Busschof and Temple were enthusiastic about the powers of moxabustion against the gout: they both considered themselves cured by the technique. Both were also scathingly critical of 'regular' European medicine, deriding it as overly devoted to theory and orthodoxy, and insufficiently interested in observation and empirical practice. But there is at least one significant difference between their attitudes towards moxabustion: while Temple expressed strong approbation of the Asian medical models and expertise which underpinned the use of moxabustion for cases of the gout, Busschof was outspokenly hostile to several prominent aspects of that expertise—particularly the notion of burning the moxas only in 'certain determined and prescribed places of the body'.[27] Thus, as I've shown above, Busschof made much play of the 'perverse custome' of hidebound Asian medical theory:

If, then, it chanceth that the Gout sits just in the place, where they are accustomed to burn, it is cured; but if it happens to be seated just one inch more or less from the place prefixed, and call for the operation of burning, they let the Patient complain and cry out, and will not succour Nature where she needs it[28]

Temple instead lauded the unanimity of Asian medical thinkers and practitioners:

I pretended not to judge of the Indian Philosophy, or reasonings upon the cause of the Gout; but yet thought them as probable as those of Physicians here; and liked them so much the better, because it seems their opinion in the point is general among them, as well as their manner [of practice] occurring; whereas the differences among ours are almost as many in both, as there are Physicians that reason upon the causes, or practice upon the cure of that disease.[29]

Why might these two men have had such different responses to an unfamiliar medical cosmology? I would argue that they are responding as much to medicine as they have seen and experienced it as they are to moxabustion in particular. Busschof witnessed first hand the medical rituals of another culture—and they looked to him both bizarre and inexplicable. He saw that culture's failures as well as its successes, and although he acknowledged the expertise of his healer, her appearance (an Asian woman) would have singularly contradicted his assumptions about what a medical expert should look like. Meanwhile, he also saw (and experienced) the failures of western medicine to treat disease in the novel tropical context: under such circumstances, over-reliance on, or overconfidence in, any established precedent could prove dangerous. Temple's perspective on medicine was, on the other hand, entirely European, where the spectacle of squabbling medical men was rapidly becoming a satirical commonplace (a view that would only strengthen in the eighteenth and nineteenth centuries). He knew of Asian medicine only second hand, as it appeared in a literature that still idolized—if perhaps for their strangeness—its successes. Drawing on these limited sources, Temple saw the persistence of gout (both as a disease, and in individual cases) in Europe as 'chiefly occasioned by the ill methods of curing it at first', and not by the nature of the disease itself. Such an understanding was inflected by his distaste for medical orthodoxy, and implied a sharp critique of 'regular' western practice as producing iatrogenic disease.

Temple and Busschof's different responses reflect their differing expectations of and interactions with non-western cultures. Early European opinions of the Far East were based largely on highly coloured travellers' tales, and translations of philosophical texts—in particular, the works of Confucius. Like many elite Europeans, Temple had drawn from this scant information an idealized vision of Chinese civilization as one which had retained the high moral and cultural standing attributed to the 'Ancients'—the civilizations of classical Greece and imperial Rome. On the other hand, Europeans who travelled to East Asia with such high expectations often lived there (or returned) in a state of some disillusionment. Over the course of the eighteenth century, their disenchantment would increase, as differences between the technological endowments and productive capacities of China and Europe became more and more noticeable. A missionary like Busschof had additional reasons to grind the axe of western medicine—it was swiftly becoming a crucial tool for conversion, and a measure of civilization (see Chapter 2).

So far, through these famous and influential accounts, I have looked at moxabustion from the patient's perspective. Unlike medical practitioners, neither Temple nor Busschof was heavily invested in any particular medical systems or theories. Thus, they focused on the process and empirical effects of the treatment, rather than on its theoretical underpinnings. There were, however, several notable accounts of moxabustion written by medical practitioners in the same period. Batavia was an extraordinary place in the late seventeenth and early eighteenth centuries. Long a geographical and cultural crossroads, Batavia was also, as Busschof's experiences suggest, a meeting place for medical cultures. Busschof mentioned, in closing his narrative, a 'Dr. Wilhelmus de Ryne, who lately is arriv'd here,' bringing with him all the latest medical news from Europe.[30] Wilhelm Ten Rhyne, like Busschof, was to prove a remarkable medical observer and cultural mediator. Ten Rhyne may even have influenced Busschof's rethinking of the gout. He was, after all, trained by Franciscus Sylvius, whose interests in fermentation and iatrochemistry must have made the idea of morbid gases developing in the sick body quite compelling. Certainly, both layman and professional came to very similar conclusions about the greater accuracy of eastern than western models of that disease (see below). However, both men also shared lingering doubts about the (predominantly Chinese) theories of the body that underpinned much of East Asia's medicine. And unlike Busschof, Ten Rhyne was a university-educated physician with a deep knowledge of Europe's scholarly medical tradition as well as its new emphasis on anatomy and physiology. He had a stake in the knowledge and structures of western medicine, and was engaged in the medical debates of the day.

Busschof encountered Ten Rhyne as the latter passed through Batavia on his way to a new posting as the medical officer of the Dutch trading mission in Japan. Once in Japan, Ten Rhyne was both observer and observed; as the sole representatives of European culture, the Dutch merchants and their entourage were studied and questioned, particularly about Western natural philosophy (what we would call science), technology, and medicine. The Dutch were swift to take advantage of this interest, and the Japanese experts who were delegated to elicit such information from them. Another avenue of communication was opened by Japanese who risked capital punishment by disguising themselves as servants to gain access to the mission, and thus the ideas and knowledge of the foreigners. Ten Rhyne and his successor, Engelbert Kaempfer, exploited both of these groups to gather as much information as they could about Japanese medicine. They certainly looked for readily transferred techniques and saleable medicines, but in this period physicians and scholars abroad also looked for expertise that could contribute to the unravelling of the processes of disease and healing. Often too, like thinkers in other fields (e.g. religion, natural philosophy, law, etc.), medics used the information and practices they discovered in other cultures to bolster one or another side of ongoing debates in the West—as in the case of gout and its treatment.

Despite their determined efforts, neither Ten Rhyne nor his medical brethren were fully able to access the Chinese medical cosmology that underlay the use of moxabustion. The language barriers were too high. Every term, every theoretical expression, every experiential fact had to be translated from Chinese (the language of medical scholarship in much of Asia) into Latin (its European analogue)—and the linguistic route of transmission was anything but direct:

I gathered and translated these [annotated body-maps] into Latin with the assistance of Iwanaga Zoko, a Japanese physician who knows Chinese, and with the assistance of Monttongi Sodaio, our interpreter, who speaks faltering Dutch in half words and fragmentary expressions. . . . I relied on Sodaio because, although not good at explaining terms, he was more experienced in medical matters than all the other interpreters.[31]

Chinese medical texts were (and are) complicated and difficult to interpret, partly because many central terms have multiple meanings. As these terms passed from Chinese to Japanese to Dutch to Latin, they lost the polysemic flexibility of their original language, and hardened into the increasingly rigid language of western medicine. The final translations were made even more brittle, as Ten Rhyne complained, by his interpreters' 'inexperience and limited vocabulary in Dutch'. Thus, he was driven to 'omit much that was written in Chinese in the original documents'.[32] Perhaps worse for the long-term survival of moxabustion (and acupuncture) than these omissions were a set of misapprehensions arising from Ten Rhyne's use of western anatomical language to translate Chinese description of the body's inner workings. These translations rendered East Asian models of the body inaccurate to the point of risibility in western eyes. But Ten Rhyne's mechanistic interpretation, though detrimental to European perceptions of East Asian medical knowledge, did allow Ten Rhyne to support a very particular model of *western* medicine. He used the observed success of moxabustion to illustrate that anatomical knowledge was not the sole basis for effective medicine. In this, he largely agreed with Busschof's critique of European arrogance and unwillingness to learn from 'pagans'. Indeed, he explicitly stated that 'The various movements of the blood must be learned through the precepts and rules as layed [sic] down by the Chinese . . . if the cure is to be undertaken according to their regimen.' However, unlike Busschof, Ten Rhyne did not believe that moxabustion had to be performed according to Chinese rules. Rather, he asserted that although anatomy had not produced moxabustion, anatomical knowledge could nonetheless substitute for the 'elaborate' experience-based precepts and detailed maps of East Asian practice. With this, he gave considerable support to the anatomists, and by extension to the emerging anatomical and physiological medicine. He took the middle ground in a debate which was then nascent and which continues even today: the clash between those who saw medicine as necessarily an idiosyncratic art, and those wished it to become a universalizing science. Ten Rhyne's compromise was typical of elite physic in his time: 'Theory furnishes laws, and experience furnishes dexterity: the best practitioner is the one who, taught and trained with both theory and experience, is a master of his art.'[33]

Ten Rhyne's successor, though almost exactly his contemporary, showed considerably less inclination to compromise. Engelbert Kaempfer was trained by Olof Rudbeck, a pioneering anatomist of the lymphatic system, and had clearly absorbed his teacher's commitment to anatomy as an explanatory mode in medicine. Thus where Ten Rhyne found much in Japanese medicine to support and extend the principles he had been taught, Kaempfer assessed the same medical system and found it deficient in the area of medicine which he had studied most closely: the circulatory system. This was doubly damaging for the prospects of moxabustion, since Japanese explanations of moxabustion depended heavily upon notions of obstructions in the healthy flows of both physical and ethereal fluids around the body. Like Ten Rhyne, Kaempfer interpreted these explanations to refer to the circulation of the blood—and consequently saw the Japanese view of the body as simply incorrect.

Nonetheless, despite his scepticism about the theory underlying moxabustion, Kaempfer was no less convinced of the technique's practical efficacy than Ten Rhyne, Busschof, and Temple. Kaempfer did not explicitly engage with the ongoing debates on gout, and ignored Ten Rhyne's westernization of Chinese explanations of the disease. Instead, he explained moxabustion's mode of operation in the light of conventional understandings of caustics, and existing European explanations of gout:

This caustick breaks the force of the saline and tartarous particles, which the too plentiful use of Rhenish wines leaves in the blood, and which, being fix'd about the joints, and particularly irritating that sensible membrane, which encompasses the bone, are the cause of gouty paroxysms.[34]

As far as Kaempfer was concerned, then, moxabustion worked like any other kind of caustic or cautery on the gout, albeit much more gently. Kaempfer did expand this very standard picture of gout to incorporate (and display) his up-to-date knowledge of the circulatory system, blithely referring to 'stagnating lymph', capillary vessels, and delicate and obscure membranes.

Kaempfer was clearly aware of Ten Rhyne's treatise on moxabustion. However, he specifically referred only to Busschof's far more popular account. He was unimpressed:

Bushofius a Minister of the Gospel at Batavia in the Indies, went too far, when he recommended the Moxa to his Countrymen in Europe, as an infallible remedy for gout. I have reason to apprehend that many a patient in Germany found himself disappointed in his expectation . . . [35]

This was a clear criticism of laymen who transgressed the increasingly well-defined boundaries of medicine. He also wryly disputed the claim that East Asian healers were in harmonious agreement on the causes and cure of disease, offering disparities in the practice of moxabustion as an example:

The Chinese and Japanese Physicians widely differ in their opinions concerning the parts of the human body which it is proper to burn with the Moxa . . . If their different opinions were brought together, I believe, that in some distempers, there would be scarce any one part of the human body left, but what some of them would single out as the most proper to be burnt with success. [36]

And even though he and Ten Rhyne were trained only a few years apart, Kaempfer already showed less regard for experience as a source of medical authority and root of therapeutic expertise. He discussed the way in which Japanese practitioners sited their moxabustion cones (and acupuncture needles) at points specific to the disease: 'These they all pretend to be well known to them by the observations of their ancestors, and by their own experience . . . '.[37] Clearly, he was unconvinced by this form of justification, and looked instead to anatomy:

The Main art [of moxabustion] lies in the knowledge of the parts, which it is proper to burn in particular distempers. . . . one would reasonably imagine that place to be the most proper which is nearest to the affected part, yet the operators frequently choose such others, as are not only very remote from it, but would be found, upon an Anatomical inquiry, to have scarce any communication with it, no more than by the common integuments. . . . I am sensible, that the most skillful Anatomist would be at a loss to find out any particular correspondence of these remote and differing parts with one another.[38]

In an earlier version of this text, Kaempfer added a revealing commentary: 'The results do not allow us to accuse all of them of deception, yet sound reasoning does not permit us to testify in defence of all of them . . .'.[39] His frustration with the theoretical intransigence of moxabustion foreshadows European responses to Chinese medicine in the next century (and within much of the medical profession, even today).

Kaempfer, like Ten Rhyne, saw moxabustion as a technique worth further investigation by Europeans. Also like his predecessor, Kaempfer understood that moxabustion incorporated not just the physical practice, but the knowledge and theories that guided it:[40]

As to the more particular rules of this burning art, they have tables printed in Chinese and Japanese characters, of which I here present the reader with one, which I endeavour'd to explain and translate, so well as the nature of the Chinese verse, wherein it is wrote, and the principles of their Philosophy would admit of. I have likewise added two Schemes, being two different views of the human body, wherein is shewn what parts are proper to be burnt.[41]

Kaempfer's adaptations of the Japanese originals neatly illustrate both his respect for Japanese medical expertise, and the limits he set upon it (see Figure 10). He had been forced by the evidence of his own eyes to accept the knowledge (authorized by centuries of experience) that certain points on the body's surface could be stimulated by

10. (FACING PAGE) 'Kiu siu Kagami', two male figures illustrating acupuncture points, from Englebert Kaempfer, *The History of Japan*, 1728. Note the very westernized appearance of the human figures and the fact that the 'Japanese' characters which decorate the page are just that: decorations. They are not legible *kanji* (ideograms). Compare to Ten Rhyne's figures (Illustrations 11 and 12), which, although westernized, still accurately depict the acupuncture channels.

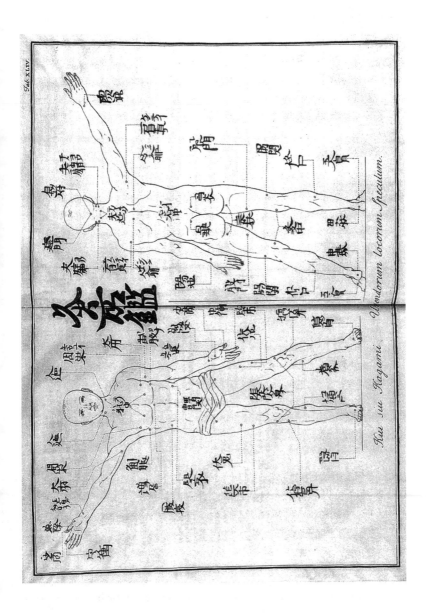

moxa to produce particular therapeutic effects. However, he clearly found the opacity of the phenomenon's mechanism frustrating. Therefore, his 'schemes' meticulously reproduced a set of the major points. However, Kaempfer refused to accept the theory that explained the power of those special points—the channels and vessels of energy flow postulated by East Asian understandings of the body. Thus where Ten Rhyne's images, though westernized, retained the *qi* channels, those channels are unmarked on Kaempfer's (see Figures 11 and 12). Moxabustion became, at a stroke, mysterious. Its basic effectiveness was unquestioned, but was also inexplicable. And where Ten Rhyne (and the laymen Busschof and Temple) had confidently expected that anatomy would in time find the structures responsible for moxabustion's remarkable effects, Kaempfer showed no such faith. Medicine was changing fast in Europe, and Kaempfer's training put him firmly on one side of the divide between older and newer medical traditions that Ten Rhyne had tried to bridge.

These four accounts of moxabustion—Busschof's first-hand report of its folk practice in Batavia and his own personal experience of its success; Temple's description of his textually mediated encounter with moxa; Ten Rhyne's maps, observations, and hard-won translations of Chinese medical texts; and Kaempfer's sceptical reinterpretations of both Japanese and European accounts—together constituted the major pathway by which the practice of moxabustion was transmitted to the West. Until the late eighteenth century, assessments of moxabustion, and to no small degree assessments of East Asian medical expertise more generally, were mediated by these texts. They are remarkable in the congruence of their descriptions of the practice itself. On virtually every count, all four describe the moxas—the pellets or cones of a fibrous vegetable substance and the use of incense to light them—and the process of moxabustion identically. The physicians' accounts are much more detailed and use some technical language, but these are differences in degree rather than kind. Therefore, we can fairly say that laymen and medics saw, recorded, and transmitted the same material practice. This fact is particularly worth noting in the case of Temple, whose moxas were applied in the absence of any first-hand witnesses to the practice of moxabustion in Asia: European doctors were able to reproduce the Asian practice drawing upon textual sources alone. Moreover, doctor and patient accounts concurred about the experience of moxabustion—its safety, its relative painlessness, and its soothing, rather than frightening, quality. All four of the documents also cite classical authorities and precedents for the therapeutic use of fire, and all pick out certain exotic attributes of the practice in Asia. These vary from volume to volume; Kaempfer focused on the ritualized gathering of the mugwort leaves themselves, Ten Rhyne and Busschof preferred to describe the 'perfumed matches'—incense sticks—with which the moxas were lit; and Temple spoke of the use of garlic to treat the moxa eschar (scorched lesion).

However, the lay authors offered little commentary on the medical theories that explained the therapy in Asia. They quite freely speculated on its mode of operation in the gout, and used its success to support alternative theories of that disease, so their silence on East Asian theories cannot be attributed to diffidence. Not were they slow to use their observation of Asian medical practitioners as a stick with which to beat the European profession—about its squabbling, its narcissism, or the brutal ineffectiveness of its therapies. It seems more likely that they were unaware of or uninterested in those theories. Their medical counterparts, on the other hand, devoted more space to East Asian medical theory than even to descriptions of the technique or instructions about its practice. But then, in a time of flux in European medicine, knowledge of another culture's medicine could offer the physicians considerable intellectual traction. Above, I've given examples of how they used these discussions to enter broader debates about development of medicine as a discipline and a profession in the West. Through the lens of moxabustion, they assessed the relative importance of anatomy and experience as sources of authoritative knowledge; they asserted the necessity of medical training to the proper performance of this powerful new therapy; they critiqued lay interventions into medical debates. The ease with which moxabustion became a Trojan horse in its narrators' internecine and intellectual battles offers another perspective on the pursuit of cross-cultural medical knowledge by medical professionals.

Moxabustion in the long eighteenth century offers an example of a moderately successful cross-cultural transmission of 'medical expertise'—that combination of knowledge (both cosmological and experiential) and practice that constitutes 'medicine' in any culture. As such it illustrates one common constellation of the factors and interests whose alignment is necessary to overcome the hurdle of cultural specificity. Medics and laypeople alike were impressed by moxabustion quite apart from its usefulness as a debating point. It was, all agreed, safe; simple to apply; and firmly buttressed by classical precedents for cautery. It offered patients a relatively painless cure for an intractable condition, and offered reputable physicians and surgeons a tool with which to challenge the hold of quacks on gout cures. The practice itself was exotic enough to be interesting, familiar enough to be domesticated.

All of these reports of moxabustion were written when the gaps between doctor and patient, and between western and East Asian understandings of the body and disease were both relatively narrow. They discuss a therapy which, while markedly exotic, was also apparently readily understood and assimilated, largely because of its material similarity to an established European therapy. To understand the importance of these factors in shaping the transmission pathways and reception of a cross-cultural medicine, therapy, or technique, it is worth looking briefly at another example, similar in the timing of its transmission, its cultural origins, its underlying view of the body, its mysterious mechanism, and its exotic appearance—but 'discovered' and transmitted to the West by physicians (indeed, by the very same physicians) rather than patients, and lacking in any immediately apparent European analogue: acupuncture. I'll argue that the difference between moxabustion's visibility and acupuncture's obscurity in the eighteenth century speaks volumes about the relative power of patient-pull (and consumer networks) and physician-push (and professional networks) as engines of 'medical multiculturalism'.

In my opinion, it also demonstrates that even misconceived notions of commonality—like the assumption that moxabustion was just another version of actual cautery—can massively facilitate the movement of medical expertise from one culture to another, at least in the initial stages.

'Meerly Upon Their Own Experience': Incorporating Acupuncture

On one of his few journeys away from the island trading-post inhabited by the handful of European traders allowed in Japan, Wilhelm Ten Rhyne observed a Japanese sailor behaving in an extraordinary manner. Writhing in pain from what Ten Rhyne diagnosed as severe colic, the sailor seemed determined to add insult to injury by piercing his own abdomen with a set of rather fearsome needles. To Ten Rhyne's utter amazement, the sailor was completely relieved by his makeshift operation, and immediately resumed his duties. Through close observation, the careful cultivation of native informants and practitioners, and the illicit acquisition of some few Japanese medical texts and images, Ten Rhyne gathered enough information about acupuncture to describe it to a European audience enthralled with that little-known nation. Neither he himself nor his audience at home appear to have regarded the technique as in any way 'quackish'. Indeed, Ten Rhyne incorporated both the technique of therapeutic needling and its apparently instantaneous effects into his explanatory model of diseases. It nicely confirmed his own pet theory that disease was largely the result of 'morbid wind' ('as many accidents may happen from wind in the lesser, as in the greater world . . . ').[42] His discussion of acupuncture as a successful treatment, however, focused more closely on instructing the trained medical practitioner—and on asserting the need for medical knowledge and expertise in applying the needles. Ten Rhyne's treatise, 'De Acupunctura', appeared in the same volume as his discussion of gout and moxabustion, and shared the same illustrations—his detailed and accurate maps of the Sino-Japanese body (see Figures 11 and 12). It was rich in exhortations to experiment with and assess acupuncture. But his incitements elicited little

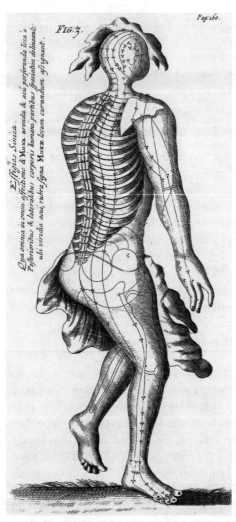

11. Chinese figure, from Wilhelm Ten Rhyne, *Dissertatio de arthritide: mantissa schematica: de acupunctura*, 1683. Note the ways in which these images have been westernized—here, the figure's 'skin' has been dissected away to hang in flaps around his skull and ribcage, mimicking European anatomical atlases, even though the *qi* channels and yang meridians have been (accurately) drawn on the body's surface.

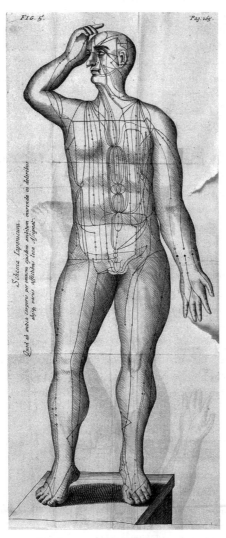

12. Japanese figure, from Wilhelm Ten Rhyne, *Dissertatio de arthritide: mantissa schematica: de acupunctura*, 1683. Here the figure's face is a western one (not unlike Ten Rhyne's own), but again the complex surface mapping of the original Japanese diagrams is retained, offering a clear, if non-western, rationale for acupuncture's effects.

reaction in Europe, and the technique was not taken up until the close of the eighteenth century. So why did acupuncture get less attention, and produce fewer responses than moxabustion?

Ten Rhyne's descriptions of acupuncture and moxabustion did not directly address the disgruntled patients of a common disease as Busschof and Temple had done. Predictably, his text provoked less response than those volumes, and was not immediately translated from Latin into the vernacular languages. However, Ten Rhyne's medical text, like Busschof's popular one, was immediately reviewed in the *Philosophical Transactions* of the Royal Society. The reviewer spent considerably more time discussing Ten Rhyne's portrayal of Japanese anatomical notions, and of the Japanese practice of moxabustion than acupuncture. His choice reflects contemporary fascination with Japan and Japanese culture: Japan had since the mid-seventeenth century proclaimed itself *sakoku*, a 'closed nation'. Only a handful of Dutch traders were allowed to enter the country at all, and native Japanese were forbidden on pain of death to communicate any information about Japan or Japanese culture to them. Reports from the few westerners with intimate knowledge of Japan were consequently of great interest to general audiences. Anatomy too was something of a closed country, and certainly a controversial one to most readers (some dissections admitted a paying audience but even they were only open to a narrow elite); hence it was likewise worthy of discussion.

It is the reviewer's emphasis on moxabustion, however, which is most revealing about the factors that either promote or stymie the cross-cultural transmission of medical knowledge. At this point in the moxabustion's own transmission process, the technique retained its attention–grabbing 'oriental' associations, but had become fairly well known among interested elites. As discussed above, moxa had been the subject of considerable public commentary following the publication of Busschof and Temple's accounts. Importantly, these discussions engaged multiple social networks: Busschof's report, as I've shown, triggered investigation in the fledgling Royal Society, while Temple's account sent a ripple of experimentation through his highly visible circle. Busschof also had a representative (his son) actively promoting the technique—and the commodities associated with it—in Europe. Moreover, moxabustion was positioned explicitly as a more pleasant alternative to existing treatments (or non-treatments) of gout, and incorporated a novel but compatible explanation of that disease. Thus it offered patients a choice, without demanding that they reject the medical cosmology they still shared with their physicians.

Compare this picture of moxabustion to the practice that Ten Rhyne named acupuncture: acupuncture was virtually unknown and had none of moxabustion's familiarity to render it accessible to lay audiences. Even the basic instrument required to perform the operation—a finely ground, very long silver or golden needle—was far from commonplace in this period (see Figures 13). The procedure he described involved penetrating (without opening) the body's surface, an act which was rare in western medicine, and when performed, highly dangerous and thus riddled with repugnant associations. His description, in fact, stressed the dangers of incautious puncturing and insisted on the importance of an anatomically informed operator. Such warnings would certainly have reduced acupuncture's appeal to the dissatisfied laymen who became such powerful advocates of moxabustion. In fact, acupuncture would come to be regarded as comparatively painless and safe, but this realization depended on direct experience of the technique in practice. Such experience was not available to Europeans until the end of the eighteenth century. Moreover, Ten Rhyne presented acupuncture as useful addition to the medical and surgical arsenal for conditions associated with cold and winds. Thus it did not benefit, as moxabustion had, from the attention garnered by being an 'alternative' to ineffective established remedies for a socially evocative disease. He deliberately addressed himself to a limited audience, and because of his long residence in the Far East, had a sparse social network in Europe itself. Neither he himself, nor any representative, returned with his treatise to promote the new therapy, and acupuncture had no readily commodified attributes to attract speculators to its support in Europe. Even with its exotic maps, its ease of operation, and Ten Rhyne's enthusiastic and informed support, acupuncture

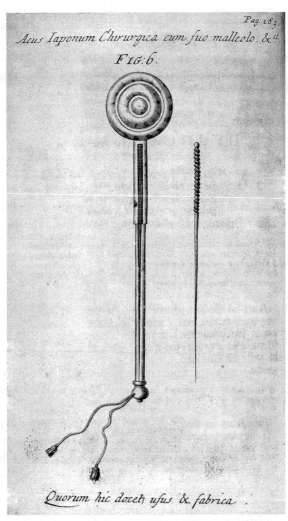

13. Japanese surgical needle and mallet, from Wilhelm Ten Rhyne, *Dissertatio de arthritide: mantissa schematica: de acupunctura*, 1683. In depicting the technology of acupuncture, Ten Rhyne was equally accurate, but clearly felt no need to render these simple instruments 'familiar' to his European audience. Note that the mallet with which the needles were tapped into the skin also serves neatly as a needle-case, rendering the technology easily portable.

as a package proved insufficient to tempt either patients or professionals to experiment.

Acupuncture got a second chance to pique the European fancy when Engelbert Kaempfer was likewise moved to report on the curious cures he witnessed there. His account of his experiences in the Far East, originally titled *Amoenitatum Exoticarum* ('Exotic Pleasures') and largely republished in vernacular as a *History of Japan*, was not a specifically medical text. Indeed, his descriptions of both moxabustion and acupuncture were offered only as appendices to the volume. They were certainly more attentive to the needs of a general audience than Ten Rhyne's accounts had been. For instance, Kaempfer reassured his readers that both of the Japanese practices he described were relatively painless:

Their very names indeed will appear terrible and shocking to the reader, they being no less, than fire and metal. And yet it must be owned in justice to the Japanese, that they are far from admitting of all that cruel, and, one may say, barbarous apparatus of our European surgery. Red hot irons and that variety of cutting knives and other instruments requisite for our operations, a sight so terrible to behold . . . are things which the Japanese are totally ignorant of. Their fire is but moderate, it hath nothing to terrify the patient . . . So likewise the metals they make use of in their operations of surgery, are the very noblest of all . . . gold and silver, of which they have needles made in a particular manner, which are finely polished, and exceedingly proper to perform the puncture in human bodies[43]

Nonetheless, like Ten Rhyne, Kaempfer addressed his description of the actual practice of acupuncture primarily to a medical audience. It is clear from his attention to detail that he intended his text to provide ample guidance for any would-be acupuncturists in his audience—as long as they were medically trained and anatomically astute:

But now to come to the operation itself . . . The surgeon takes the needle near its point in his left hand, between the tip of the middle finger, and the nail of the forefinger, supported by the thumb, and so holds it towards the part which is to be pricked, and which must be first carefully examined, whether it be not perhaps a nerve, then with the hammer in his right hand, he gives it a knock, or two, just to thrust it through the hardish resistent [*sic*] outward skin.... The precepts and rules of this pricking art are very different, with regard chiefly to the hidden vapours, as the supposed cause of the distemper. Hence, when the operation is to be performed, a careful and circumspect Physician must determine with all his attention and judgement, where and how deep they lie.[44]

Like Ten Rhyne before him, Kaempfer did acknowledge that Japanese laymen and women often self-punctured with perfect success—'Even the common people will venture to apply the needle, meerly [*sic*] upon their own experience'. But even this statement carried a rider to warn off the experimentally inclined European laity: 'taking care only not to prick any nerves, tendons, or considerable blood vessels'.[45] Given the unfamiliarity of the technique, its tools, and even of the idea of deliberately running a needle into one's own flesh, acupuncture would hardly have seemed an easy option. As the next chapter will detail, radical changes in the focus both of practitioners and patients were required to bring acupuncture into the medical spotlight.

Conclusion

By the late eighteenth century, after a century of reports on moxabustion in Asia and later its use in Europe, it had become a familiar, if not a common, therapeutic practice. Moxabustion was best known in France and ironically, given the importance of William Temple's essay on the technique, least known in Britain. It retained faint connections with its East Asian origins, which critics of the technique often emphasized in conjunction with its erratic efficacy. Several complained also about moxabustion's painfulness, though even its opponents admitted its mildness compared to the 'regular' European techniques of actual or chemical cautery. Moxabustion's proponents—many of whom were prominent surgeons who had seized upon moxabustion to extend the therapeutic scope of their discipline—meanwhile, had broadened the term and restructured the practice of 'moxabustion'. They experimented with more readily available substitutes for the vegetable fibres used for moxas in Asia;

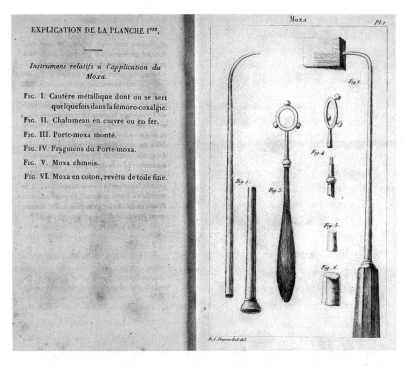

14. 'Instrumens relatifs à l'application du Moxa', from Baron D. J. Larrey, *Récueil de Mémoires de Chirurgie,* 1821. Tools were not typically used in Chinese and Japanese applications of moxa, but better suited emerging western norms of practice.

and they invented or endorsed tools with which to apply the burning material. These tools effectively westernized the process of moxabustion, both reducing the amount of direct physical contact between patient and practitioner, and eliminating disturbingly foreign elements of the treatment (e.g. the use of incense-sticks to light the moxas, worm-casts as a base for the burning fibres, and raw garlic as a post-operative ointment) (see Figure 14). Likewise, moxabustion was reinterpreted theoretically in terms of contemporary scientific preoccupations with imponderable fluids:

[The Moxa] appeared to me to communicate to the parts, along with a corresponding mass of caloric, a very active volatile principle which cottony substances furnish, when they are in a state of combustion. The irritation and excitation resulting from the combination of these two products . . . are gradually propagated to the most deep-seated parts, so as to restore the action of the weakened or paralyzed nerves, and to stop the progress of the morbid cause, seated in any particular part.[46]

In the practice of moxabustion too, efforts were made to reduce its dependence on exotic models and maps of the body. Crucially, westernized moxabustion relied on the practitioner's knowledge of general anatomy and individual patient-histories (e.g. the location of a particular patient's first twinges of gout) to determine where to burn, rather than on the mapped sites traditionally related to different symptoms and patient-groups in Chinese practice (which had, in any case been much diluted and distorted in the transmission process).

Over the course of the eighteenth century, the value of familiarity in facilitating cross-cultural transmission seems indisputable. Moxabustion after Kaempfer did not challenge western models of the body or medical practices; however, neither did it change them. Instead the technique was largely absorbed into the medical mainstream, losing its identity as it was westernized and mechanized. Having been so successfully likened to caustics and cautery, when those techniques went out of fashion, so too did moxabustion. Acupuncture, on the other hand, had no European analogue to launch it into the marketplace. Nor did it capture the attention of a group of patients, as moxabustion had captured gout sufferers. I have found no records of acupuncture being practised in Europe before the 1780s. But then, its mysteriousness actually became an advantage. Because acupuncture remained unclaimed and unexplained—indeed precisely because in the quest for familiarity it had been mistakenly analogized to the western practice of bleeding by Europeans who had never seen acupuncture practiced by experts— it became the subject of investigation and experimentation by a French clinician investigating the therapeutic efficacy of bleeding. The next chapter explores medicine in the nineteenth century, and the parallel rise of both 'scientific' and truly 'alternative' medical systems. Acupuncture, as I will describe in Chapter 3, rose and fell in the interstices between these opposing medical poles.

2

HEALTH AND 'THE NEW SCIENCE'

Given the prevailing indifference of late eighteenth- and early nineteenth-century European medicine to Chinese and Indian medical theories, it is perhaps ironic that this period also saw the rise of both mesmerism and homeopathy. Each of these systems drew heavily on ideas of manifest, but ethereal vital energy, energy that was depleted or defective in unhealthy bodies but which could be channelled or activated to restore a natural state of health. Both systems therefore postulated a model of the animal economy remarkably similar to those that underpin Chinese and Indian medicine, and practices like *qigong* and yoga. Their dependence on intangible and invisible forces seems strongly counter to the prevailing materialist trends of medicine and science in the period, and today both are regarded as alternative medicine. However, in the late eighteenth and nineteenth centuries, homeopathy and mesmerism made strong claims to scientificity, were championed by medical elites, and were popular first with precisely those educated consumers who also avidly pursued the natural sciences.[1]

Mesmerism and homeopathy were strikingly popular across the nineteenth century and into the twentieth, even as the ideals and institutions of medical orthodoxy were being forged in their turbulent wake. Their proponents and postulates met with responses ranging from ecstasy to abhorrence; neither system could be seamlessly assimilated, yet both produced 'legitimate' medical offspring. Taken together, a study of the origins, rise, and decline of these now-heterodox or 'alternative' European approaches to healing will allow us to assess the distinctiveness of western responses to cross-cultural medical expertise and systems. Were European responses to Chinese medicine, for example—whether positive or negative, assimilative or purgative—responses to its foreignness or simply to its difference from established medical beliefs and models?

Sensational Science: Mesmerism and Medicine, 1775–1900

In 1775, Anton Mesmer (1734–1815), a trained Viennese physician, proclaimed a new basis for medicine. Mesmer was certainly a showman; but he was also a scientist, and by the standards of the day, a fairly proficient one. Steeped in scholasticism by his medical education, he was also stimulated by the new scientific styles and knowledge emerging around him—in particular by the new 'fluids' or substances that were regularly reported in the burgeoning scientific press: electricity, phlogiston, caloric, magnetism, and others. He claimed to have discovered a genuine natural substance, which he called 'animal magnetism'. It was a 'subtle fluid' in both the classical and the Newtonian senses—Mesmer himself likened it to gravity and *aether* as well as the newly discovered 'galvanic fluid', electricity. By 1784, Mesmer confidently answered the question 'What is magnetism?' with the statement that 'It is the property which bodies have of being susceptible to the action of a universally distributed fluid, a fluid which surrounds all that exists and which serves to maintain the equilibrium of all the vital functions.' He might almost have been quoting from classical Chinese or Ayurvedic descriptions of their respective vital energies.

The possibility that such a substance might exist in the human body first occurred to Mesmer in response to an older work, which suggested that the body, like the seas, might feel the gravitational pull of the planets—that human tissues were subject to 'tides'. Indeed, Mesmer also defined animal magnetism as 'the property of the animal body that renders it sensitive to the action of heavenly bodies and of the earth.' Mesmer was convinced that the presence and proper action of the magnetic fluid (like those of *qi* and *ojas*) ensured health. Conversely, a sick person might be cured of nervous conditions by the stimulation of his or her mesmeric fluid, or by a dose of the substance transferred to them by an individual super-endowed with animal magnetism, by reason of moral and physical superiority. Mesmer himself was such a person naturally, but less fortunate individuals could build up their reservoirs of animal magnetism through efforts of will. Alternately, he discovered that a sick individual could benefit from the pooled (or stored) magnetic energy of a group of merely normal, but healthy people.

After an initial rebuff in Vienna, Mesmer set out in earnest to popularize his discovery. In 1778, he moved to Paris and began by offering treatments to those who attended his clinic-salon in Paris. He called his new, quasi-Masonic establishment 'The Society of Harmony', and gave it the motto, 'All things in due weight and measure.' As his choice of motto suggests, Mesmer sought scientific credibility as avidly as popular acceptance, and believed profoundly that the 'magnetic fluid' would eventually be quantifiable. His salon was dominated by an enormous 'tub' filled with water and magnetic material (mainly metal bars and iron filings), which Mesmer considered to be a mesmeric magnet, charged with the collected fluid of his own and his patients' animal magnetism. From the periphery of this tank projected metal handles. His patients grasped these handles during treatment, while Mesmer willed the tub's stored energy into their bodies, triggering the mesmeric 'crisis' or trance.

Supported by a wave of interest in the new discovery of electricity, Mesmer's technique for a time produced good results; patients proclaimed the success of his cures, and the scientific establishment looked on bemusedly. Most of Mesmer's successful cases were among middle- and upper-class women, whose attendance at his clinic was due as much to fashion and politics as to medical complaints. These patients, surrounded by acquaintances and fellow sufferers, were fixed by the intense gaze, and sometimes stroked by the wand, of Dr Mesmer. If a 'crisis' was produced, the individual might faint, cry out—perhaps with pleasure, perhaps in pain—or even fall into a fit. It was this peculiar, unpredictable, and highly personal interaction between a male physician and predominately female patients, combined with a taint of political radicalism, which troubled the medical and scientific establishment. Indeed, Mesmer's discovery was publicly discredited by the findings of an Académie de Médecine commission, led by a panel of the scientific great and good appointed by Louis XVI in 1784. Despite the reaction which Mesmer could produce in his clients—and which he was able to train others to produce as well—neither a physical explanation for 'animal magnetism', nor any substance analogous to the 'magnetic fluid' could be found. But mesmerism had not been targeted for investigation because it was scientifically suspect—many established medical techniques lacked experimental evidence of their mechanism and few had more than anecdotal/empirical evidence of efficacy—Mesmerism was investigated because it existed in an atmosphere of sexual tension and titillation. Nor was Mesmer disgraced by the collapse of his theory in the face of science; rather, he was driven out of Paris by the unstated assumption that his therapeutic invention threatened the chastity of his predominantly female patients, and depended on their mental weakness.

Mesmer's personal fall from grace did not result in the disappearance of animal magnetism from either the popular or the medical stage. Nor was the 1784 verdict of the French Royal Commission regarded as conclusive; mesmerism continued to spread, crossing the English Channel alongside such innovations as the stethoscope. By the 1820s and 1830s, the practice of mesmerism and its ostensible cause, the substance 'animal magnetism', was once again the subject of earnest and eager investigation. In France, Laplace considered 'animal magnetism' if not a proven, then at least a possible action of, or influence upon, the nerves. Moreover, the Académie de Médecine, which had derided mesmerism in the 1780s, finally sanctioned it (after a five-year investigation) in 1831.

In London, the Cambridge-educated John Elliotson, newly minted Professor of Practical Medicine at University College London, was an enthusiastic proponent. Like Mesmer, he believed fervently that science and experiment would vindicate the medical practice of mesmerism and would discover a physical mechanism for its sublime effects. He felt that animal magnetism and the phenomena it produced would finally give radical physiology the tools necessary to make it a science of the living, rather than

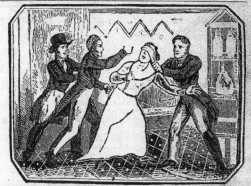

A female Patient being blindfolded, to undergo an operation.

15. 'A full discovery of the strange practices of Dr Elliotson', illustrated title page of anonymous 1842 pamphlet published in London. Not only was Elliotson marked for his early and enthusiastic adoption of medical mesmerism, but for his equally enthusiastic adoption of the early nineteenth century's most scandalous garment: the trouser—regarded as far too form-fitting for decency. Note the prominent mention of 'female patients', 'secret experiments', and 'curious postures'.

the dead. More importantly, animal magnetism seemed to Elliotson and his reforming medical colleagues to prove the materiality of the mind and will, and thus to place them firmly within medicine's sphere of influence. He therefore offered a series of public demonstrations of his own mesmeric practices and patients, demonstrations that were in the end to destroy his reputation and career within the growing medical establishment.

Elliotson's experiments were dramatic spectacles, performed on and through the living bodies and captive minds of some men, but principally young working-class women, charity patients in the University College Hospital (see Figure 15). These women were, in the eyes of animal magnetism's proponents and experimentalists, moulded by the magnetic power into reliable scientific apparatus or machinery. Initially, Elliotson used them to demonstrate the properties of animal magnetism (for example, that it was transmitted in straight lines, like rays), and the powers it had over (and could released in) the human organism. Thus, his young subjects were hypnotized via mirrors, lifted weights beyond their strengths, imitated his unseen movements, and saw through closed containers, or even (and most controversially and for the medical profession threateningly) the human body—the latter enabling these medically untutored and apparently unsophisticated girls to diagnose illnesses and even predict life or death.

While Elliotson and other proponents of animal magnetism excitedly discussed the amazing strengths and heightened senses bought about by the magnetic influence, and their therapeutic and scientific potential, their adversaries scrutinized the experiments, the girls, and their doctors alike for fraudulence. The 1830s and 1840s were a critical period in the professionalization of medicine. Medical reformers and traditional elites were already at each other's throats, fighting for control over the future of organized medicine. Meanwhile, friction was growing between doctors and patients as the former sought ever greater social status and authority, and the latter clung on to their traditional role as primary readers and interpreters of their own bodies. In this heated atmosphere, the idea that individuals—and particularly working-class women—could become the arbiters and apparatus of medical experiment was potentially subversive, and provocative in the extreme. In 1837, Thomas Wakley, editor of the *Lancet* medical journal, finally took direct action to address the growing controversy and damaging rumours. Wakley, through his prominent, often-cantankerous, and highly readable weekly journal, had been among Elliotson's strongest supporters, and a consistent advocate of medical and social innovation. However, he was also a chief advocate for a reformed and scientific medical profession—and in his view, Elliotson's experiments, and in particular their dependence on by-now unpredictable and all-too-human 'subjects', were threatening the standing of both science and professionalism in medicine. He set out to expose Elliotson as a dupe and the girls as frauds. In doing so (through a series of experiments performed in his own home in front of a panel of witnesses, half of whom had been chosen by Elliotson and half by Wakley himself), he ended Elliotson's once-dazzling career, and his patients' sojourn in the medical spotlight (as well as their treatment at University College Hospital).

After the Elliotson debacle and others like it, few individual practitioners were willing to support mesmerism publicly. Professional bodies and their individual members aggressively attacked the technique as quackery and its remaining supporters as sleazy charlatans or gullible fools. This high-handed approach sometimes backfired. Harriet Martineau, a noted author, traveller, political essayist, and in the later years of her life, invalid and mesmerism enthusiast, reflected in her controversial *Letters on Mesmerism*:

The systematic disingenuousness of some Medical Journals on this subject, and the far-fetched calumnies and offensive assumptions with which it is the regular practice of a large number of the Faculty to assail every case of cure or relief by Mesmerism, looked very much as if they were in conflict with a powerful truth, and as if they knew it.[2]

In desperation, she had herself been mesmerized to treat an internal illness, and described the sensation as one of a 'clear twilight' falling across her and slowly melting away the objects before her. She also felt heat, oppression, sickness, and disorder of the stomach.

Unsurprisingly, given such powerful experiences, mesmerism remained a popular topic of debate and demonstration, and mesmerists and their opponents cluttered the Victorian lecture circuit. Mesmeric societies spread across Britain, some cities supported mesmeric infirmaries (though all had closed by the 1860s), and access to mesmeric journals was widespread.[3] Every drawing room of consequence devoted time to 'the New Science'; mesmerism, through the power of mesmerists from all walks of life to entrance and control their 'betters', became an argument for political and social reform. It was used to argue for the reality of the supernatural, for the scientific basis of some forms of traditional medicine, and for the meaningfulness and validity of a truly popular science.

As mesmerism resisted all attempts at eradication, doctors and surgeons quietly—even secretively—began to test its limits themselves, noting mesmerism's empirical effects but denying all the while the existence of any 'magnetic fluid' (see Figure 16). Martineau, as a prominent and prolific author, started to receive letters on the subject once her support for experimentation with the technique became known:

There is a remarkable uniformity in the letters I have received from medical gentlemen from various parts of the country, each believing himself to be almost the only one who has ventured upon the practice of Mesmerism, either from scientific curiosity, or from the failure in particular instances of all other means,—each having two or three valuable cases to report,—and each suffering under the experience or apprehension of ill-will from his professional brethren from the hour of his avowing any belief in Mesmerism.[4]

In 1842, one aspect of this experimentation burst into the public sphere, when a respectable Nottingham surgeon collaborated with a local mesmerist to amputate a patient's leg under 'mesmeric anaesthesia'. The patient lay quietly throughout the gory operation, and later reported no pain. It is worth remembering that at this point, pain control in surgery was limited to the dulling effects of drink; all operations were performed with the patient conscious and often physically restrained. Indeed, like the 'laudable' disease of gout in the preceding century, the pain of surgery was believed by many to

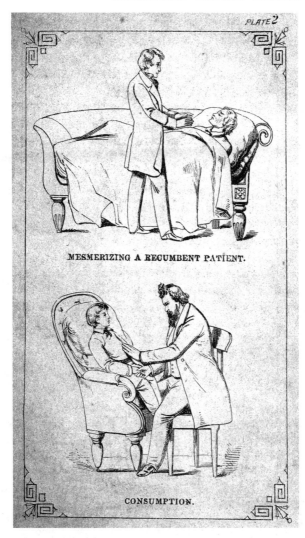

PLATE 2

MESMERIZING A RECUMBENT PATIENT.

CONSUMPTION.

16. Treatment of consumption and tuberculosis by mesmerism, from William Davey, *The Illustrated Practical Mesmerist*, 1854. Not all images of mesmerism were dramatic or scandalmongering. These far more conventional images present the mesmerist as a decent family practitioner—and present mesmerism as a valuable therapy for serious physical ailments.

be healthy and an essential part of treatment. As one scandalized clergyman (himself the brother of a surgeon-mesmerist) reported: 'The Royal Medical and Chirurgical Society of London permitted Dr. Copland, without a word of disapprobation, to declare that, "pain is a wise provision of nature; and patients ought to suffer pain while their surgeon is operating; they are all the better for it, and recover better."' Dramatically, the outraged minister asked his readers: 'How can medical men in this country justify their heartless apathy in regard to Mesmerism?'[5] Surgical patients, like their gouty predecessors, were certainly less convinced of the therapeutic benefits of pain; thus mesmerists' claims to have vaulted this hurdle presented surgeons and the orthodox profession at large with a dilemma. Should they adopt the technique they had so bitterly castigated to free surgery from its brutal past, or should the feat of painless surgery too be rejected as simply another example of mesmeric fraud and collusion between weak or scheming patients and their mesmeric masters? It may seem impossible to us even to imagine feigning calm or sleep while experiencing an amputation, or the removal of a cancerous breast, but many argued that this was exactly what patients were doing. In Britain, the debate raged around the question of the reliability of the patient's own experiential testimony, until it was replaced in 1846 by debates over the value and safety of ether and other chemical anaesthetics (sometimes in comparison with the safety of its mesmeric analogue).

Ether was promoted very deliberately by the medical profession to combat the popularity of mesmerism. And it did have benefits for the busy medical practitioner: it was predictable and speedy in its actions; it acted independently of the patient's will or volition; it was under the sole control of the administering doctor. Otherwise, it had few advantages over mesmeric anaesthesia—and none from the patient's perspective, since it was more dangerous, produced nasty side-effects (including an alarming number of fatalities), and was perhaps even less explicable. Nonetheless, with the staunch support of the orthodox medical community, it succeeded in displacing its mesmeric rival not merely from surgery, but from medical practice almost entirely. The mesmeric technique itself, stripped of its claims to a material basis and often trading under the untainted name of hypnotism, continued to be applied in private homes and public lecture theatres in pursuit of knowledge or pleasure. For a time it persisted even in doctor's surgeries as the death toll of chemical anaesthesia continued to climb. And despite its European decline, mesmerism was not everywhere banished from public medical debate. As Chapter 4 details, it thrived in imperial India, alongside orthodox western medicine, and another competing European medical system: homeopathy.

The 'Law of Similars': Homeopathy and the Rise of 'Alternative Medicine'

In 1810, Samuel Hahnemann (1755–1843), a university-trained but highly dissatisfied German physician and translator of medical texts, declared his discovery of two new medical 'laws'. The first of these principles—called 'the law of similars' after Hahnemann's famous phrase '*similia similibus curantur*' (like treats like)—was, he asserted, based on his own careful observation and self-experimentation. Hahnemann reported that those substances which *caused* the symptoms of a particular disease in healthy person would *relieve* those symptoms in their sufferers. The experiment which had convinced him of this had actually been constructed to determine the effects and action of an established medicine: in 1790, Hahnemann deliberately ingested cinchona bark—rich in quinine—and experienced in consequence symptoms of the malarial fevers which that drug famously cured.

Hahnemann's second principle (and the most derided aspect of homeopathy both in the nineteenth century and today) was the 'law of infinitesimals'. Unlike the law of similars, the law of infinitesimals was rooted in theoretical reasoning on the nature of disease, rather than in observation or experiment. Essentially, Hahnemann (like many other physicians, before and since) believed that disease sprang not from a simple breakdown in the bodily mechanism—which would demand similarly mechanical treatment: for example, purges to vent impurities, or emetics to remove blockages—but from disturbances of the body's ethereal vital force. Thus treatments needed to act on the metaphysical, rather than the corporeal, level. This rationale was, of course, not unlike that offered by mesmeric healers to explain that system's more than physical effects. Hahnemann argued that the therapeutic potency of a medicine in this metaphysical realm increased as the material medicinal substance itself was mixed, diluted, and refined:

For its own special purpose and by its own special procedure . . . homeopathy develops the inner, spirit-like medicinal powers of crude substance to a degree hitherto unheard of, and makes all of them exceedingly, even immeasurably penetrating, active, and effective. . . . This remarkable transformation of the properties of natural bodies through the mechanical action of trituration and succussion on their tiniest particles . . . develops the latent dynamic powers previously imperceptible and as it were lying hidden asleep in them. These powers electively affect the vital principle of animal life.[6]

Hahnemann claimed to have derived his 'laws' and the therapeutic system built around them through reasoned experiment, rather than through either scholarly theorization or full-throttle speculative empiricism alone. However, his 'new science' was clearly attuned to ongoing debates in the medical community—debates with which his work as a translator of eighteenth-century medical texts would certainly have made him familiar. Most importantly, Hahnemann's system tapped into an increasingly widespread belief among medical professionals and consumers alike in the *vis medicatrix naturae*—the healing power of nature. In the *Organon der rationellen Heilekund* (first published in 1810, translated rapidly and widely, and generally referred to in English as the *Organon of Rational Healing*, or just the *Organon*), he argued that within all living bodies resided an innate healing power: 'In the state of health the spirit-like vital force (*dynamis*) animating the material human organisation reigns in supreme sovereignty. It maintains the sensations and activities of all the parts of the living organism in a harmony that obliges wonderment.'[7] Similarly, emerging models of disease as 'self-limiting' bolstered his system. These models proposed that diseases had a natural course through which they would inevitably progress, ending in a 'crisis' during which the patient's 'dynamis' or vital force would either be exhausted or be restored to a state of healthy balance.[8] In combination, these two ideas suggested that the most effective therapeutic strategy was to strengthen the body for its inevitable ordeal, and to assist nature in reaching the 'crisis' before the body had been exhausted (a doctrine that would subsequently underpin the mid-nineteenth-century orthodox reformers' turn towards therapeutic nihilism). Hahnemann had no doubt that his method of treating like with like would surpass and supersede orthodox methods, which he termed 'allopathy'—'treatment with opposites'—and derided for opposing nature's own healing process and thus depleting the body. But he intended to go beyond merely assisting 'diseased nature' down her own 'very imperfect' path.[9] Hahnemann reasoned that the artificial diseases reliably and briefly induced by his 'proven'—experimentally tested—medicines more powerfully engaged the patient's vital force. The strong symptoms thus artificially induced 'extinguished' the weaker (but more persistent) effects of the natural disease, then disappeared as the medicines left the patient's system: 'By giving a remedy which resembles the disease the instinctive vital force is compelled to increase its vital energy until it becomes stronger than the disease which, in turn, is vanquished.'[10]

Another area of heated debate among Hahnemann's medical contemporaries was the question of disease classification (or 'specific disease'). Could physicians distinguish with certainty one disease from another and treat it (in accordance with whatever explanation of its causation was then current) or could they be sure only of the individual patient's set of symptoms? In other words, did diseases exist as specific and knowable entities separate from the bodies in which they were expressed, or was every patient's disease experience unique and particular? The way in which a practitioner answered these questions had ramifications for every aspect of medical practice. If a practitioner believed in specific diseases, he (and in orthodox practice, it was all but inevitably a he) would strive to identify and treat that disease in increasingly standardized ways. However, practitioners dubious of specific disease identifications and standard treatments would tailor their treatments to individual patients and sets of symptoms. Men and women, adults and children, rich and poor, city-dwellers and country folk, sickly and hale, gluttonous and abstemious, pillars of virtue and slaves of the flesh—each would need slightly or radically different therapies. Since Hahnemann was suspicious of medical claims to be able to explain and identify diseases (although not necessarily of the notion of specific disease), he hedged his bets. His new medical system focused very closely on individual constellations of symptoms, rather than on what he regarded as largely speculative disease entities. Indeed, Hahnemann argued that the symptoms *were* the disease: 'Illness is the sum of its symptoms.'[11]

Given this assumption, it was imperative that homeopathic practitioners elicit from their patients a complete and detailed description of their entire disease experience. However, for any given constellation of circumstances and symptoms, homeopathy claimed that it could produce a proven specific remedy. Thus although homeopathy was based on two fairly straightforward principles, its practice depended on an elaborate complex of factors:

We only require to know, on the one hand, the diseases of the human frame accurately in their essential characteristics and their accidental complications, and, on the other hand, the pure effect of drugs; that is, the essential characteristics of the specific artificial disease they usually excite, together with the accidental symptoms caused by difference of dose, etc. and by choosing a remedy for a given natural disease that is capable of producing a very similar artificial disease we shall be able to cure the most obstinate diseases.[12]

Despite Hahnemann's blithe 'only', homeopathic practice clearly demanded a substantial burden of prior knowledge, especially as few known drugs had yet been tested on healthy individuals. In particular, homeopathic treatment depended heavily on a detailed patient history, and on precise patient-reporting of symptoms. Homeopathic practitioners could not rely exclusively on their own reading of the patient's body, because it was the patient's *experienced* illness (and personal circumstances) that determined the appropriate remedy. A homeopathic physician might spend several hours on the initial consultation, simply in taking the patient's history:

The patient details the history of his sufferings. Those about him tell of what they have heard him complain, how he has behaved, and what they have noticed in him. The physician sees, hears, and remarks by all his other senses what there is of an altered and unusual character about the patient. He writes down accurately all that the patients and his friends have told him in the very expressions used by them ... When the narrator has finished what he would say of his own accord, the physician then reverts to each particular symptom and elicits more precise information.[13]

As with mesmerism, homeopathy's emphasis and dependence upon patient testimony presented a sharp contrast to trends in orthodox practice, where doctors were increasingly interested in uncoupling diagnosis from the 'subjective' experience of illness. Through technology and technique, regular medicine was struggling to declare independence from the patient; homeopathy instead reinforced the role of the patient as a partner—albeit often unwitting and in need of expert guidance—in the diagnostic process. Hahnemann explicitly notes that the patient's 'own account of his sensations is most to be trusted' adding only the parenthetical caveat '(unless he is feigning illness)'.[14]

Homeopathy was also dependent on physicians' willingness to serve as their own experimental alembics (again, demonstrating a degree of comfort with subjective evidence which was disappearing from 'regular' practice); on the thoroughness and precision of their reports when 'proving' drugs; and on the continuous pursuit of such experiments. In this combination of attributes, homoeopathy united two already diverging strands of medicine—the rationalist system-building of learned medicine with its balance of universal 'laws' and individual experience; and the rising empiricism of 'scientific medicine' with its hypotheses and experiments. It is perhaps this combination of familiarity and novelty that rendered homoeopathy so pernicious in the eyes of orthodox medical professionals—and so very attractive to medical consumers.

Like Hahnemann himself, medical consumers in the early nineteenth century were far from satisfied with the therapeutic offerings of the medical profession, and in particular with the prevailing fashion for dangerously emphatic treatments. Not only were their testimonies increasingly discounted, but their bodies—vulnerable sick bodies, at that—were subjected to newly punishing measures in search first of diagnosis, then of cure. 'A disgust of medicine' was hardly surprising when that medicine might entail (as, famously, in the case of George Washington's last illness):

two copious bleedings; a blister applied to the part affected; two moderate doses of calomel [a mercury-based emetic]; an injection . . . which operated on the lower intestine . . . another bleeding, when about thirty-two ounces of blood were drawn, . . . vapours of vinegar and water . . . ten grains of calomel . . . repeated doses of emetic tartar . . . blisters applied to the extremities and a cataplasm of bran and vinegar to the throat.[15]

Patients were regularly bled to syncope (unconsciousness), cupped, and scarified. As well being bled through these general or local means, they were puked, purged, and poisoned; in some common diseases (for example, syphilis), patients were treated with mercury until their teeth loosened in their jaws. Medicated enemata offered another route to rebalancing the body's input and output, particularly in conditions such as hysteria, and disorders of the menses. And of course, there were the leeches. One American patient, Emily Mason, wrote to her sister of the treatment she was due to receive for facial pain: 'Today, I am threatened with leeching—Don't you envy me having those sweet little worms in my mouth?'[16]

These harsh therapeutic tools formed the backbone of a rising medical trend: 'heroic medicine'. Although all of these methods and medications had long pedigrees in western medicine and were accepted by doctors and patients alike, the first third of the nineteenth century saw their usage taken to the very extremes of human endurance in search of medical 'activity'. In assessing the rationale behind such apparently horrific treatments, it is worth remembering that although orthodox doctors in this period knew considerably more about the internal structures and workings of the body than their predecessors, their new knowledge had not yet led to any novel therapies. Even Jenner's much lauded innovation of vaccinating with cowpox against the much more deadly smallpox did not constitute a cure, merely a far safer and often more effective preventive. So medical practitioners found themselves in the invidious position of making greater claims to authority based on their improved ability to describe the actions of disease upon the body, without being any better at explaining the origins of, or actually treating, disease. Moreover, their new knowledge, dependent as it was largely upon pathology, required investments at both the personal and professional level. Not only did individual practitioners have to spend both time and money acquiring pathological training (and moreover to do so at the risk of their own health, given the dangers of accidental self-contamination in the charnel house); but the profession too had to invest its capital as a humane art in the distasteful practices of human dissection (and while familiarity may have blunted our distaste for dissection, the controversy which has, as recently as 2003, greeted public exhibits of the dissected body—whether glossed as art or education—suggests that it remains just beneath the surface). Homeopathy represented an entirely different vision of medicine, then, in very fundamental ways. It was deliberate and gentle; it did not aim for or produce instantaneous or dramatic effects on the human body. It was, at least as framed by Hahnemann, profoundly anti-materialistic, and rooted its model of disease not in ever-more minute examinations of the physical body, but in attentive observations of the experiential one. Like mesmeric physiology, homeopathic knowledge was self-declaredly rooted in the living body, not the dead—specifically the bodies of all its 'proving' practitioners.

From its origins as a critique from within the boundaries of elite German medicine, homeopathy spread rapidly to the rest of Europe, and accompanied the waves of German immigrants to the United States. In France and Britain, but especially in the United States, it found fertile soil, well prepared by the therapeutic excesses and monopolistic ambitions of orthodox medicine.[17] Indeed, homeopathy—with its emphasis on mild, easily self-administered, and highly portable drug therapies—was particularly well suited to the exigencies of a geographically dispersed, necessarily self-sufficient, and generally wilful population. And Jacksonian American, culturally and politically marked by a rejection of elitism and professional claims to exclusive knowledge, was already shrugging off early attempts by its nascent medical profession to regulate the practice of medicine, and make it a preserve of the 'regularly trained'.

The chronology of medical regulation in America during this period demonstrates both the surging but often thwarted ambitions of medical practitioners, and the close relationship between culture, politics, and medical pluralism. Before the 1830s, medicine in the United States largely followed the professional model established in Britain. Medical societies were founded (the first, in Boston, in 1736), as were medical schools (beginning with the College of Philadelphia in 1765). Shortly thereafter, medical societies began to promote binding codes of practice which discriminated against 'irregulars'—lay and religious healers, itinerant practitioners, proponents of non-canonical medical systems, and anyone else claiming to practise medicine in the absence of training either through apprenticeship with an established doctor or surgeon, or in a medical school. By 1830, the United States had twenty-two medical schools, and thirteen states had passed laws which allowed local medical societies to license medical practitioners. Although these laws carried little force, they did raise the status of 'regulars' and gave them the exclusive right to sue for the payment of their medical bills. But these first steps towards an established orthodoxy were already being undermined by Jacksonian scepticism, by the continued proliferation of other medical systems—many rather better suited to the American context—and by the burgeoning industry of medical certification. New York journalist Mordecai Noah captured the changing mood of Jackson's America in 1830, when he stated bluntly: 'medicine like every useful science should be thrown open to the observation and study of all.' Meanwhile, medical degrees were becoming accepted as equivalent to the licences issued by professional societies. This provoked a boom in highly profitable proprietary medical schools—essentially 'diploma mills', with low standards and even lower admissions requirements.

Between 1830 and 1840 in the United States, 6800 new doctors graduated from such schools, to the disgust of their better-trained colleagues and medical consumers alike. As one critic writing in a medical journal complained:

It is very well understood among college boys that after a man has failed in scholarship, failed in writing, failed in speaking, failed in every purpose for which he entered college; after he has been dropped down from class to class, after he has been kicked out of college; there is ONE unfailing city of refuge—the profession of medicine.[18]

'Regular medicine' soon found itself caught in the proverbial cleft stick: on one hand, the mood of American society was staunchly anti-elitist, and equally strongly in favour of the dissemination of all useful knowledge and skills by every available means. On the other, the nascent educational institutions and regulatory systems that were intended to justify the privileges and authority claims of the medical profession were often themselves manifestly corrupt. Medical deregulation swiftly followed. Between 1830 and 1850, all but two states repealed their laws restricting medical practice to regularly qualified practitioners. Thus the United States came to offer an untrammelled and unrestricted medical frontier to practitioners of all therapeutic stripes, and consumers were left free to assess the merits of competing systems and practitioners as they saw fit.

In 1847, elite US practitioners founded the American Medical Association (AMA) explicitly to combat the 'irregulars', who were rapidly gaining ground and establishing their own institutions and journals; and equally explicitly, to eradicate, regardless of system, all those who, as noted physician, Worthington Hooker, put it in 1849, practised 'medicine as a trade instead of a profession, and [studied] the science of patient-getting to the neglect of the science of patient curing'. The AMA sought to restore the credibility of the 'regular' profession partly by closing the wounds caused by competition between orthodox practitioners. It regulated minimum fees, barred consultation with irregulars, and banned grubby advertising. However, the Association faced a long and uphill struggle. Its homeopathic opponents were often 'regularly' educated and better

qualified—and they offered their well-heeled clients a far more palatable therapeutic course (an American journalist in 1848 was inspired
to verse: 'The homeopathic system, sir, just suits me to a tittle | It
proves of physic, anyhow, you cannot take too little').[19] Meanwhile,
for their poorer or rural adherents, homeopathists established
homeopathic dispensaries and even mail-order homeopathy medicine chests—highly suitable for life on a frontier chronically under-
served by medical practitioners of any system. These institutions and
businesses alike persisted well into the twentieth century, despite
major challenges like the 1910 *Report on Medical Education in the United
States and Canada*, known universally as the Flexner Report after its
author Abraham Flexner (a noted educational reformer, but not a
doctor). Ostensibly Flexner's famous survey of American medical
education supported no system, but only 'modern' medicine: 'Prior
to the placing of medicine on a scientific basis, sectarianism was, of
course, inevitable. Everyone started with some sort of preconceived
notion, and from a logical point of view, one preconception was as
good as another. . . . Modern medicine has as little sympathy for
allopathy as for homeopathy.' However, his findings set a new
standard for medical education in which basic sciences, laboratory
training, and hands-on clinical education reigned supreme. Few of
the homeopathic medical schools (and indeed few 'regular' institutions) met this standard, or could raise the funds necessary to improve their facilities. Many went under; but the last surviving
homeopathic medical school (the Hahnemann Medical College
and Hospital of Pennsylvania) only finally severed its ties to the
homeopathic system in the 1950s after over a century of teaching.

In Europe too, homeopathy was no short-lived fad; it was the
system of choice for the British upper classes and gained royal
patronage amongst Victoria's many offspring (patronage that homeopathy still retains today, with London's Homeopathic Hospital
still operating under the Queen's warrant). As regularly trained
William Kingdon (1789–1863) reported in an 1827 speech to his
medical brethren, patient demand was essential to the spread of
homeopathy—and perhaps the most important force in the creation
of converts from within the medical profession itself.

My most profitable business is with gentlemen in the city, whose object it is to have their maladies attended to, if possible, without interference with their usual avocations—men whose minds are enlarged by education and occupations,—whose habit is industry, and whose fortune is the profitable occupation of their time, equally removed from the indolent and the luxurious, who readily catch at novelty for amusement, and the ignorant and unlettered, who are easily caught by any appearance of mysticism. Such men as these have been requiring me, for the last eighteen months, to try, as they call it 'Homeopathy,' at which I only smiled incredulously, and I fear, contemptuously. The reiteration of such applications, however, and from men in whose judgment and veracity I had confidence, seemed to demand from me some investigation of the subject; and desirous to set about it in the most fair way, I sought an introduction to Dr. Quin, of whom I had heard most honorable report.[20]

Conversions, or even speculative dabbling like this, were a blow to the heart of orthodoxy. Like the United States, nineteenth-century Britain also suffered from proprietary medical schools, over-competition among medical practitioners, and popular contempt for large portions of the orthodox profession. The luxuriant growth of British homeopathy was therefore no less threatening and loathsome to its orthodox profession. The pages of the *Lancet* and the *British Medical Journal* (*BMJ*) were filled with bitter diatribes against homeopathists, and indeed against their clientele—castigated as faddish, ignorant, deluded, self-indulgent, and of course, those old favourites, hysterical and hypochondriacal. And in this furnace of fear and loathing was the orthodox profession forged. The competition offered by the homeopathic system drove 'regular' practitioners—previously absorbed by the internecine warfare between elite and general practitioners—to organize and identify as one profession. Moreover, homeopathy's commercial and therapeutic successes also forced major changes in orthodox medical practice. As the prominent and well-regarded physician Sir John Forbes grudgingly noted in 1858:

The favourable practical results obtained by the homoeopathists—or to speak more accurately, the wonderful powers possessed by the natural restorative agencies of the living body, demonstrated under their imaginary treatment—have led to several other practical results of value to the practitioners of ordinary medicine.[21]

Despite scoffing at homeopathy's 'imaginary treatment', Forbes carefully enumerated the beneficial effects of inter-system competition:

[I]t has tended directly to improve their practice, by augmenting their confidence in Nature's powers, and proportionately diminishing their belief in the universal necessity of Art, thus checking that unnecessary interference with the natural processes by the employment of heroic means, always so prevalent and so injurious. It has thus been the means of lessening, in a considerable degree, the monstrous polypharmacy which has always been the disgrace of our Art—by at once diminishing the frequency of administration of drugs and lessening their dose.[22]

Even as he argued that homeopathy merely took credit for Nature's own miracle cures, Forbes acknowledged the reciprocal weaknesses of orthodox practice: 'unnecessary interference' and 'monstrous polypharmacy'.[23] Reviewers applauded Forbes's text, though few were as forthright as Forbes himself about the impact of homoeopathic successes on regular practice.

Homeopathists themselves were only too aware of their impact on orthodoxy. One homeopath observed allopathic borrowings with an air of amused superiority:

[T]he 'sweeping over us' of homoeopathic knowledge . . . made *patients* less tolerant of bloodletting, and so doctors had to give it up; and as they found that diseases did better without it, they had to alter the teachings of their text books accordingly, and they had to invent some other reason for their altered practice, and the 'sweeping over us of cholera' or 'the change of type of disease' served to save their dignity . . . [24]

Others expressed indignation at the allopathic pillaging of their pharmacopoeia, and unacknowledged 'plagiarism' of their practices of expectant medicine; and minute doses. Their hostility was only strengthened by continued attacks on homoeopathy from the allopathic camp. Naming prominent 'regular' names with abandon, one homeopath wrote, 'Black, Thorowgood and many others recommend bits of homeopathic practice without mentioning the hated word. Wilks filches from us while he abuses us.'[25]

In Britain and Germany, as in the US, medical professionals at the mid-century fought hard to re-establish a single orthodoxy and to imbue it with social, legal, and moral standing. As in the US, their efforts, beginning with organization (the British Medical Association was founded in 1832, and was intended, like its US counterpart, to fight orthodox corruption and quackery alike), self-regulation and the raising of educational standards, and building on the successes of the emerging 'germ theory' did meet with considerable and growing success. However, homeopathy's powerful lay constituency and its elite corps of well-educated, well-organized (the British Homeopathy Society, for example, was founded in 1843, only a decade after the orthodox British Medical Association), and upper-class practitioners, if unable to resist some marginalization, nonetheless successfully prevented 'allopathy' from being enshrined in law as exclusively synonymous with 'medicine'. Indeed, homeopaths were able to force an amendment to the 1858 Medical Act (which established a regulatory body to supervise 'regular' medical education, and the annual publication of a Medical Register of qualified practitioners), which prevented medical licensing bodies and medical schools from discriminating against 'irregulars' so long as they were medically qualified. As in the US, the British government had no stomach for restricting the free trade in medical thought—or commodities.

Both homeopathy and mesmerism presented themselves initially as radical innovations within established medicine. Only as they were squeezed out by orthodox hostility did these systems reposition themselves as 'alternatives'—as challengers to the medical system they had intended to reform. The two systems shared not only a belief in imponderable forces or energies that could be turned to the task of curing; they also shared certain aspects of practice. Both, of course, were highly time-consuming, homeopathy because of its elaborate system of provings and detailed case histories, mesmerism because of the need to condition the patient to respond to the mesmerist's gaze and touch. Both also depended heavily on subjective, experiential data, either from the mesmerized patient or from the homeopathist's experience of proving. Perhaps worst of all in the eyes of the orthodox profession, mesmerism and homeopathy both went around the medical establishment, to address the patients themselves. One well-known medical convert to mesmerism, James Esdaile (see Chapter 4) bitterly protested the lack of a 'Free Trade in medical knowledge', after a paper describing his mesmeric practice in India, initially solicited by a respectable medical journal, was suddenly rejected.[26] Denied the freedom of the medical press, Esdaile stubbornly published his article himself as a pamphlet. This fits well with his approach in a book-length version, in which he urged patients themselves:

to exercise their common sense and sober judgment in determining for the doctors the matter of fact; and if the community decides that it is really a remedy of great efficacy, that there is no resisting the proofs in support of it, that to know nothing about it is no recommendation to a medical man; then Mesmerism will assume its proper rank as a remedial agent . . . [27]

Esdaile was himself regularly qualified, and far from desiring a free medical marketplace; he wanted the practice of mesmerism to be firmly 'lodged in the hands of those who alone should practice it': other orthodox doctors and surgeons. 'Instead of doubting and dogmatising about Mesmerism, I would earnestly entreat my medical brethren to put it to the test by personal experiment.' What Esdaile in fact wanted was for consumer pressure to force the medical profession to change its stance on mesmerism—to render it orthodox. Unfortunately, although mesmerism could be smuggled into the private sickroom, it was harder to dismember than homeopathy; consequently, it could not be selectively (and by subterfuge) integrated with orthodoxy in the same way that homeopathy's most consumer-friendly attributes and practices had been.

Despite their shared features, homeopathy and mesmerism were far from similar in other ways, and produced quite different effects on the medical profession. In Europe, mesmerism perpetuated sexual hierarchies and in India (see Chapter 4), hierarchies of race, even as it challenged hierarchies of class. Homeopathy, on the other hand, was instrumental in opening the medical profession to women (and to a lesser degree, non-whites) particularly in the United States. This openness was not entirely disinterested. Doctors had long recognized that women were the family decision-makers in matters of health. Noting 'the growing aversion to large doses of strong and disagreeable medicine among the more liberal and progressive elements in society', one contemporary commented that 'many intelligent women had become tinctured with the heresy of Homeopathy and gave a preference to the physician who would prescribe or administer their milder and pleasant remedies'.[28] As this American author (married to an early orthodox female physician) observed, this offered an opportunity for women of either medical sect: 'conformity to the demands for mild remedies gave the women doctors access to many families whose views were in accord with the reform movements that recognized the growing interest in enlarging the sphere of woman'.

John James Garth Wilkinson's 1855 booklet *War, Cholera and the Ministry of Health*,[29] promoting the use of homeopathy in the British war effort in the Crimea, aptly illustrates the benefits that accrued to homeopathy by its radical inclusion of women as professional colleagues. As he argued for the special feminine suitability of the practice of medicine, Wilkinson sounded themes that would have been very familiar to his audience:[30]

In all respects one half of medical practice belongs to Homoeopathic woman. Only note her qualities. The first of these is intuition, the bird's eye of her ever busy love.... Were this intuition fixed and educated, it would readily pass into stable medical sight. Her fine sense animated by this, might soon eclipse the corresponding organism in the man in several fields of diagnosis.... [31]

Homeopathy had much to gain from recruiting women. For example, as he recited these stereotypes of femininity and invited women into the homeopathic profession, Wilkinson also claimed for homeopathy the purity that had become a 'feminine' trait. And by likening allopathy to slavery, he sought to harness the campaigning morality that had emerged as such a powerful weapon in abolitionism:

Woman ... is the pillar of Homeopathy; she first saw the horrors of the old system in her own nursery among her loved ones; she has first experienced the blessing of the new. It was she that emancipated the slave: it will be she that ultimately rescues the Briton from the crooked and venomous darts of physic. She will then enter upon one of her own callings from which she has too long been excluded.[32]

In one area, the recruitment of women was in fact necessary: homeopathy, having marketed itself in particular to women as a means by which to spare themselves and their children from the horrors of heroic medicine, needed female bodies on which to 'prove' new homeopathic drugs for the treatment of 'female complaints'. By the standards of the profession, the provers of drugs had themselves to be trained and skilful observers: ideally, homeopathic doctors.[33] Wilkinson also emphasized the status of homeopaths as 'an independent middle class' of healers, not a bad prediction of origins of the women in his target audience.[34] And like many others in this period, he claimed for homeopathy the honour of effecting woman's emancipation from the domestic sphere: 'Hahnemann, without having that end in view, has done more than anyone else perhaps towards the emancipation of woman, by providing her with a field of the most humane and artistic usefulness, in which her beautiful powers can expand . . . What then may we not augur for medicine when an entire better half is added to it?'[35] Women too benefited: through sectarian medicine, particularly homeopathy, many of the first generation of female medical practitioners gained access to the medical profession as a whole.

Despite the challenges of 'scientific medicine' and the wholesale reform of the institutions and practices of orthodox medicine, homeopathy entered the twentieth century in strength. In Britain, it continued to have the support of the royal family and much of the social elite as well as a large middle-class following. British homeopathy differed from its US counterpart in its enduring reliance on medically qualified 'converts' as practitioners, and on a well-to-do client base. But eight cities had their own homeopathic hospitals, which treated charity patients as they trained generations of medical students. And the working poor could choose, in 1900, from thirty-five recognized homeopathic dispensaries, while homeopathic remedies were even more widely available for self-medication.

Although the number of homeopathic doctors continued to fall, their institutions survived and were indeed included first by the 1911 National Insurance Act (which insured all working men, and paid approved institutions and practitioners for their care) and subsequently the National Health Service (NHS).

The integration, finally, of homeopathy into orthodox medicine, under the auspices of the NHS was not without controversy, pain, or its own particular ironies. Many homeopathists were intensely sceptical of the intentions and outcomes of integration; the Scottish branch of the British Homeopathic Society adopted in 1941 a resolution expressing their anxiety about the effects of state control, and calling for the national society to 'ensure the right of medical men to independent judgment in matters of treatment' (though it is only fair to note that many non-homeopathic doctors were expressing exactly the same concerns about state intervention in therapeutic decisions).[36] Others were convinced that exclusion from the NHS was a far greater threat to the long-term survival of their beloved system. An editorial in the *British Homeopathic Journal* in 1944 took an accommodating approach:

There is a tendency for all minority movements, be they political or otherwise, to assume a self centeredness which is apt to result in the obscuration of the highest aim of general endeavour . . . the homeopathic body one feels is not free from this taint. . . . [Some] wittingly or unwittingly adopt the very attitude which it would seem can but antagonize even those who are not unsympathetic to the homeopathic point of view . . . The discoveries of medicine are free to all. So should the homeopathic view be proffered. Not with a superior air that this or that is 'the *whole* truth and there is not other!', but with a gentler assurance that we find this or that seems to give us better results and inviting enquiry and trial by experiment . . . To shut one's eyes to the discoveries of chemotherapy . . . is, one feels, foolishness. The 'pure' homeopath so called is a crank living in his own little cell. The complete physician is he who endeavours to know all, and knowing all, to choose what is best for the patient.[37]

Another correspondent took a slightly different approach to the process and goals of integration: 'I would view with regret any tendency to segregate Homeopathy more than is necessary for the preservation of our hospitals, because that is not the way of progress. Rather let us infiltrate into ordinary medical practice until Homeopathy (and I refer to the "pure" brand) is understood and given its proper place in the healing art.'[38] The focus of homeopaths on the preservation of the remaining homeopathic hospitals, and the establishment of homeopathy as an independent specialty was effective—as far as it went. But homeopathy in general practice struggled from the outset to survive under the geographic limitation of patient pools, and time-constraints imposed by NHS practice, and many homeopaths chose to stay in their more lucrative and flexible private practices instead.[39] In 1950, the Faculty of Homeopathy Act formally recognized homeopathic teaching, research, and practices, but homeopathic training—the lifeblood of any speciality—was denied public funding by the old enemy, the British Medical Association (through its offshoot, the British Postgraduate Medical Federation). In the end neither the sponsors not the sceptics of homeopathy on the NHS could have predicted the revival of homeopathy's fortunes and popularity of the 1970s and 1980s— in part due to changes in the funding of entirely orthodox general practices. Not only was the system taken up eagerly by consumers and lay practitioners rediscovering the *Organon*—it also became once more the subject of clinical and scientific experimentation (see Conclusion).

Medical consumers and providers often draw a strict division between orthodox medicine—in the West, typically high-tech, hospital-based, officially sanctioned and steeped in science—and 'alternative', 'complementary', or 'quack' therapies. But this distinction is fluid and contingent: the boundary between 'orthodox' and 'heterodox' must be actively policed by both lay and professional authorities if it is to remain stable. The cases of mesmerism and homeopathy illustrate how that boundary was established and sustained over time. In subsequent chapters, I will examine the ways in which notions of heterodoxy and orthodoxy have been applied to cross-cultural medical practices.

3

'THE CHINESE HAVE A GREAT DEAL OF WIT'

The Scientific Revolution sparked a re-evaluation of natural knowledge just as waves of European exploration were rapidly expanding it. In the same year, 1543, Copernicus argued for the reorientation of the cosmos from geocentric to heliocentric in *De revolutionibus orbium coelestium*, and Vesalius remapped the human body in *De humani corporis fabrica*. Between them, these two works threatened the foundations of scholastic knowledge, the former by challenging the underlying assumptions of both classical philosophy and Christian theology; the latter by undermining the dominant Galenic models of the humoural body. Scholasticism scarcely crumbled under their weight; it took a century and a half for the changes which historians collectively term 'the Scientific Revolution' to become mainstream. But observation (initially astronomical and anatomical, and later in physics, mathematics, and physiology) moved rapidly to the heart of European efforts to understand their natural world. Francis Bacon codified the new approach—based on inductive reasoning from both experiment and observation—in his *Novum organum*, published in 1620. Ancient cosmological models, systems of interpreting the world based on ideas and ideals about it, were to be replaced by knowledge gained directly. Tellingly, the motto of Royal Society of London, perhaps the archetypal institution of this period, was 'Nullius in verba'—'On the word of no one'. The goal of this new knowledge, as well as its epistemology, was fundamentally different: instead of Christian stewardship of nature, Bacon famously declared 'I come in very truth leading to you nature with all her children to bind her to your service and make her your slave.'[1]

The eighteenth-century Enlightenment drew heavily on this kind of 'natural philosophy' and its emphasis on a 'mechanical' universe (one operating according to knowable rules rather than to achieve unknowable ends, to slightly oversimplify the idea of Aristotelian 'final causes') as an alternative to theology. Similarly, Enlightenment thinkers deployed experiment as an alternative to experience or scholarly authority. With the declining power of tradition and revelation as sources of social and political authority, established social structures were, at least theoretically, under threat and subject to re-examination. If social roles, rights, and responsibilities were to be determined rationally, then new and compelling reasons for societies' inequities—for the subjugation of women and slaves, for the power of hereditary elites, for the disenfranchisement of the lower classes and non-white races—had to be sought. Meanwhile, the battle between empiricism and scholasticism (a battle in which each side claimed experience as its talisman, but differed on whether 'experience' meant first-hand observation or classical precedent) absorbed much medical attention. As we saw in Chapter 1, the front lines had already been drawn as information about acupuncture and moxabustion was in transmission from the Far East to northern Europe. Busschof and Temple, as patients with little investment in the status of scholarly medicine, unsurprisingly valued their own experiences above the precedents of scholarly medicine. Ten Rhyne, classically trained but immersed in an entirely separate medical tradition, was aware of and mediated between the two camps; he argued for a balance between practice and theory, empirical experience and scholarly art. Kaempfer's response however, signalled the coming changes: he chose to filter his observations of Japanese medicine through a systematic, speculative empiricism, in which the value of the empirical or experimental observation was determined largely by the status of the observer as knowledgeable, well trained, and 'philosophical'—or, as we might put it, 'scientific'. Moreover, this ideal informed observer (or 'modest witness') was assumed to be a European, a fact that would have a heavy impact on responses to the medical expertise and systems of other cultures.

By the close of the eighteenth century, as the emergence of homeopathy and mesmerism suggests, storm clouds shrouded the medical horizon, portending change but not predicting its trajectory. They sprang from the convergence of eighteenth-century revolutions in the social contract, the rapid emergence of new groups and types of medical consumers, medical trends whose own origins were rooted in seventeenth- and eighteenth-century shifts in epistemology (that is, in the ways and places we seek knowledge, and the systems we use to assess and validate it). In this chapter, I will scrutinize the nineteenth-century consequences of this perfect social and ideological storm in the culture of medicine. Two medical innovations—each in their different ways characteristic of the period—will provide lenses through which to focus on specific aspects of nineteenth-century medicine: the hybrid practice of acupuncture in the West, and the fiercely heterodox (but firmly European) practice of homeopathy. Looking through the eyes of both doctors and patients—the most immediate contrivers and consumers of medical innovation and change—I will assess the impact of shifts in the sources of medical authority. These in turn signalled and enforced increasingly broad divides between lay and medical understandings of the body and disease. Alongside and integral to these changes came the definition and ossification of the previously fluid boundary between the categories of orthodox and heterodox medicine—themselves unstable. None of these shifts, so crucial to the shape of medicine as we see it today, were either natural or inevitable: they had to be 'sold' to all participants in the marketplace of medical culture.[2]

Sir John Floyer's largely positive assessment of Chinese medicine (discussed in Chapter 1) at the beginning of the eighteenth century already suggested the trend of European attitudes towards non-European thought. In explaining his efforts to reconcile Chinese and European models of the pulse, he commented, 'the Asiatic have a gay luxurious imagination, but the Europeans excel in reasoning and judgment, and clearness of expression.'[3] Without explicitly ranking those two virtues, Floyer nonetheless made it clear that reason trumped imagination, at least in the sphere of medicine. By

1735, the Jesuit J. B DuHalde, compiler of the *Lettres Édifiantes* and author of the hugely influential *Description Geographique, historique, chronologique et physique de l'Empire de la Chine* (translated in 1741 as *Description Of The Empire Of China*) expressed even stronger doubts as to the very nature of Chinese intelligence and learned knowledge:

'Tis true, we must acknowledge that the Chinese have a great deal of wit: But then is it an inventive, searching, profound wit? They have made discoveries in all the sciences, but have not brought to perfection any of those we call speculative, and which require subtilty [*sic*] and penetration.[4]

Since China was then seen as the pinnacle of non-western civilization, DuHalde's scepticism about Chinese speculative and analytical ability was applicable by extension to all non-European 'science'.

The increasingly ambiguous intellectual status of medicine during this period is also revealed in DuHalde's text. After his critique of Chinese science, he admitted that the differences between Chinese and European medicine were less pronounced, at least in practical terms: ''Tis certain, that the Chinese are not less skillful in the cure of diseases with their medicines than the European physicians.' DuHalde then praised Chinese pulse diagnostics at some length. However, he attributed their discovery of, and skill with, this 'piece of knowledge, so very important for the sure application of medicines' not to scientific prowess, but to 'long experience, and a yet longer application of patience, *to which the phlegm of a Chinese can with less difficulty submit than the vivacity of an European*'. Clearly the prestige of experience was fading in European eyes—now it was a matter of stolid phlegm, not inventive flair—as newer (and faster) methods for acquiring knowledge of the body arose from the deadhouse. But DuHalde ended his discussion of Chinese medicine with a telling comment:

We may no doubt be surprized to find the Chinese (who are so little versed in the science of anatomy, which is the most important part of physic for discovering the causes of diseases) reasoning as if they understood it. They supply what is wanting in this part by experience . . . *And when all is done, no more sick persons die under their hands than do under those of the most able physicians in Europe.*[5]

DuHalde and his peers were by no means blinded by science: they were well aware of the mismatch between the accuracy and the applicability of European medical knowledge.

Abbé Jean-Baptiste Grosier (1743–1823) makes much the same point even more sharply in his *A General Description of China*:

It is true that they [Chinese physicians] never use dissection, and that they do not even open the bodies of their dead; but if they neglect to study nature in dead subjects, which always leave much to be guessed, it appears that they have long studied living nature with profound attention, and with advantage. Living nature may, perhaps, not be impenetrable to an observation of three thousand years.[6]

Medicine, then, was not yet 'scientific', and anatomy—though intellectually important—had not yet proven its practical worth, and was therefore received with some ambivalence. European medicine could not claim the absolute superiority over its non-western analogues that had already been achieved by Europe's more abstract sciences. But experience was clearly regarded as a poor second best in terms of explanatory efficiency, and its use was validated by ancient precedent and contemporary expedience, not modern practice. Grosier subsequently drew a telling analogy: 'The Egyptians did not permit the opening of dead bodies, yet it was from their sacred books that Hippocrates derived the greater part of his knowledge.'[7] In other words, just as the Egyptians provided the foundations for Hippocrates' far more important medical speculation, so the Chinese might offer raw observational 'knowledge' but not understanding or analysis. That would be supplied by the western physicians who considered themselves Hippocrates' natural heirs.

Acupuncture from Experiment to Empiricism

Europeans saw themselves as uniquely able to stand outside culture, tradition, and the gross claims of embodiment; these qualities of self-alienation were, in turn, regarded as essential for the production of 'objective' and 'reasonable' knowledge. Of course, this definition excluded not only non-Europeans, but also other groups: women,

children, the uneducated poor—and patients. The late eighteenth
and nineteenth centuries brought, as we saw in Chapter 2, increasing hostility among medical professionals to patient testimony as a
source of authoritative information about the (sick) body. The new
empiricism had little room for the unobservable data of the disease
experience. Instead, doctors who espoused it focused on new tools
for assessing the quanta of illness and cures. Sir John Floyer, of
course, had early touted his pulse watch as a more precise and
practical means of interpreting the pulse, that precious indicator of
internal bodily states—and one that did not depend so heavily on
long experience or deep knowledge. He had been ahead of his time,
but by the first decades of the nineteenth century, instruments were
beginning to seize the medical centre-stage. With the publication of
Laennec's *On Mediate Asculation* in 1819 and subsequent expansions
and popularization of its principal claims, the stethoscope too
became a potent symbol of a future in which medical access to
the internal body would be through their own, technologically
enhanced senses, unmediated by the patient, 'objective' and therefore authoritative.

This was the 'empiricism'—specific, quantitative, materialist—
which would come to dominate elite medicine by the end of
the eighteenth century, and mainstream medicine by the mid-
nineteenth century. But it could not be applied with equal rigour
to every aspect of medical practice. Some practices, treatments, and
beliefs were far too central to both doctor and patient expectations
to be put rashly to the empirical test. One such treatment was
bleeding. Long a mainstay of western medicine, both as a preventive and a cure, bleeding was, if anything, growing even more
prominent in 'regular' medicine as the nineteenth century began.
It had an extensive classical pedigree and highly visible empirical
effects—yet its benefits had never been experimentally verified, or
even (in modern times) systematically explored and categorized. In
1809 the Bordeaux Academy of Medicine addressed itself to this
lacuna (without challenging the merits of the practice itself), by
offering a prize to the best respondent on the subject of therapeutic
bleeding:

What are the advantages, and particular properties of the diverse manners of drawing blood, and their disadvantages? What principles should direct the use of one or the other? . . . And what are the proper considerations upon which to determine the choice of parts from which it is appropriate to make these evacuations?[8]

A young physician named L. V. J. Berlioz took up the challenge. Among the methods of bloodletting he included in his initial survey of the 'sanguinary evacuations' was acupuncture.[9]

Over the course of his investigations, Berlioz came to regard acupuncture highly for a very particular range of ailments. He also became aware that acupuncture was not properly to be considered a form of bleeding. Nonetheless, that acupuncture was even considered in a study on the relative merits of different styles of bloodletting offers a clear indication of how little known the technique was, even a century after its initial transmission. We know that considerable information about the technique was conveyed to Europe by Kaempfer and Ten Rhyne, well-trained medical observers, and that they offered clear indications that acupuncture, if performed properly, did not involve bleeding. So how did Berlioz come to include acupuncture in his list? His error offers a powerful demonstration of the European drive to familiarize the exotic in medicine, as a prelude to assimilating or discarding it. But while this tendency speeded the acceptance of moxabustion (and promoted its subsequent integration and virtual disappearance), it proved damaging to acupuncture's reception.

Both moxa and acupuncture were stripped—partly in transit, and partly on arrival—of the body/cosmology that explained their use and efficacy. Moxabustion, by its apparent resemblance to actual cautery, was supplied with an alternative explanation that interfered relatively little with its practice. No such simple comparison was available for acupuncture, at least not as Ten Rhyne and Kaempfer described the practice they had observed. However, their assertions that Asian physicians pierced the body with needles without drawing blood was regarded as patently unlikely, if not impossible—and were therefore dismissed, particularly in medical circles. The London-published *Medical and Physical Journal*, for example, scathingly remarked:

[W]e are told that deep punctures are first made in the body, upon which balls of moxa are burnt. These punctures are made with needles, and the skill is to determine their number and depth. We are rather startled by the information that these *deep punctures* are not to draw blood: but this rests on the authority of the Abbé Grosier, and we fear the prop is but slender.[10]

Once such contrary evidence had been erased, European practices of local bleeding could provide the much-desired analogue for acupuncture. By the 1740s, this transformation had been completed. In medical dictionaries, the new 'encyclopaedias', and other durable resources of 'regular' medicine (sources which were frequently consulted by interested laypeople as well as practitioners), acupuncture was regularly defined as method of therapeutic bleeding:

Acupunctura. *Acupuncture*. It signifies a particular way of bleeding, by making a great many small punctures with a sharp instrument, made of gold or silver. It is much practiced in Siam, Japan, and other Oriental nations, in all parts of the body, even on the bellies of women with child. *Heister*.[11]

Unfortunately, as a method of bleeding, acupuncture was found wanting. Established methods of phlebotomy (the medical term for bleeding), like venesection (opening a vein with a lancet), leeching, cupping, and scarification (applying a spring-loaded fixed array of blades to the body, thus swiftly making a number of shallow wounds) released large amounts of blood in a short space of time, producing striking changes in the appearance and state of the patient. These changes were predictable and readily explained within the humoural and physiological models of the body shared by both practitioners and patients. Needle-pricks, on the other hand, only slowly released very small amounts of blood—certainly not enough to produce the dramatic effects which were part and parcel of bleeding's appeal and rationale. In fact, the effects of acupuncture, as reported by its proponents abroad, could only be assessed through patients' descriptions of their internal sensations. Moreover they were not easily explained by anatomy or physiology, and bore no relation to those produced by European modes of bleeding. Worse, doctors were themselves, and expected their patients to be, at best amused and at worst horrified by the treatment.

One professor at the University of Edinburgh, for example, described the use of acupuncture on the hip as a treatment for sciatica as 'the conversion of the "seat of honour" into a pincushion'.[12]

As a method of bloodletting, then, acupuncture was a dead loss in the eyes of medical practitioners and consumers. Largely ignored after Ten Rhyne and Kaempfer's reports, it faded into near-invisibility. But it was precisely this invisibility—the fact that acupuncture had no particular constituency—that rendered it so available for exploration by investigators like Berlioz. Acupuncture could be subjected to the new regime of experimental assessment, and no one stood to lose if it failed the test. In fact, the failure of such an exotic technique would only prove the superiority of rational western medicine over the 'pompous pathology' and medical traditions of the East. But as Berlioz discovered, acupuncture seemed empirically efficacious, particularly for muscular pain, and nervous conditions. Patients felt better and their symptoms disappeared after acupuncture treatment. When the Société de Médecine de Paris repeated the provincial society's questions in their own competition in 1812 and again in 1813, Berlioz submitted his research not just on techniques of bleeding but also on acupuncture. His essay took an Honourable Mention, and he published it under the auspices of the two Societies in 1816.

Like Busschof's account of moxabustion in the late seventeenth century, Berlioz's study of acupuncture in the early nineteenth struck the right note at the right time and in the right place. Elite Europeans in the dawning Enlightenment had been titillated by the exotic backstory of moxabustion, tempted by its promise to safely treat the intransigent (and culturally resonant) gout, and trusting of Busschof's credentials as a reporter—he was, after all both an educated European and had himself experienced the treatment. Similarly, Berlioz's cachet as one of the new French 'clinicians', his restrained empiricism, and his focus on nervous complaints suited the rather different needs and tastes of the early nineteenth-century medical marketplace. Paris had become the centre of the medical world, a hub for medical students from across Europe and North America, who thronged its great hospitals and exploited the abundant 'clinical material' and pathological specimens those institutions provided. A later proponent of acupuncture, Robley Dunglison, demonstrated the importance of these resources in establishing the viability of medical and surgical innovations: 'In the hospitals of St. Louis, La Pitié, and Hôtel Dieu, of Paris, acupuncturation was practised some thousands of times, and in every case, according to Guersent, without the occurrence of any thing unpleasant.'[13]

The emergence of new models of the body (and disease) also stimulated interest in acupuncture. These new hypotheses were based on increasingly materialistic interpretations of humouralism; they retained the assumption that the body was a system in a state of dynamic equilibrium, but anticipated and sought the physical substrates of that fluid system. Acupuncture's mysterious effects and mode of operation—taken in conjunction with its clear empirical success—raised questions to which experimentalists hoped their new models would provide answers. For example, could the Chinese and Japanese practice of treating certain conditions by performing acupuncture at sites far from the location of the pain be explained by the new imponderable fluid 'electricity'? If so, the ancient practice of therapeutic needling might point the way for a revolution in medicine. Such speculation placed acupuncture among the first therapies to be examined in terms of its electrical potential. Similarly, clinicians and experimentalists hoped that the strange power of the metal needles might finally provide a diagnostic test of whether a patient's ailment sprang from 'a disorder of the nervous system' or from somatic disease. This distinction had, of course, been made by earlier medical generations, but rose to prominence as a focus of medical interest in part because of increasing scepticism of patient self-reporting ('he [the patient] will seldom tell the truth, and perhaps never the whole truth', grumbled William Buchan in 1796[14]). Berlioz himself pursued both of these interrogative strands, speculating that acupuncture

'acts by stimulating the nerves, or by restoring to them a principle of which they [were] deprived through the effects of the pain. . . . Very likely, the communication of galvanic shock produced by Volta's apparatus would increase the medical effects of acupuncture.'[15]

As a vector for experimentation, and a site for testing broader medical hypotheses, acupuncture proved far more captivating to medical audiences than it had been as merely another exotic medical import. However, its origins were still too interesting to medical consumers (and too problematic for medical professionals) to be entirely erased. Berlioz responded to this dilemma by introducing acupuncture in terms of its exciting past, but simultaneously denying Chinese and Japanese physicians any intellectual credit for discovering or refining the technique:

The savage peoples living in the torrid and temperate zones were . . . in the habit of marching almost nude when they went into combat. They [therefore] experienced the necessity of imprinting on their bodies some particular signs, which . . . enabled them to identify themselves. The operation which they practised to that end having been by chance done on injured parts, the resultant relief ensured its repetition in analogous circumstances. The need for signs graven on the skin having ceased with the progress of civilization, and the pricks seemingly procuring the cure only of a tiny number of maladies, the usage was lost in most nations. *This remedy has been conserved only by the Chinese and the Japanese, their neighbors, where all the first institutions are sacred.* . . . It is from these people that we take the method of acupuncture.[16]

As has often been the case when Europeans have borrowed medical or scientific expertise from non-western cultures, the Chinese were painted merely as chance discoverers and rote preservers of ancient knowledge, not its skilful creators. Berlioz and his cohort did not refer to or reproduce the Chinese body map; nor did they acknowledge or (publicly) experiment with its system of specific points.

In the absence of the perplexing body maps and explanatory notes so painfully translated by Ten Rhyne and Kaempfer, acupuncture was reintroduced to the western world by its Parisian exponents as a stand-alone technique. In other words, 'acupuncture' in this western incarnation ostensibly entailed no more and no less than puncturing the living body with a needle. While both lay and professional audiences continued to associate acupuncture with its Asian roots, these ties were ornamental. Acupuncture as practised in Paris made no appeals to yin, yang, *qi*, or a system of channels and vessels linking the body's organs with its surface; nor did its supporters claim that acupuncture was a 'specific' for any particular diseases. Rather they pointed to its empirical success in individual cases, and in certain categories of complaint (particularly nervous and chronic pain). Framed in this way, acupuncture neither conflicted with nor challenged established understandings of the body and disease, even though it could not be fully integrated with them. Thus, although acupuncture's mechanism remained mysterious to western medicine—and indeed is unexplained in biomedical terms today—it was not dismissed as quackery. Even tentative analogies drawn between acupuncture and animal magnetism (another, more controversial 'imponderable fluid' of the day) did not drive the practice out of 'regular' hands (though proponents of the technique were active in disputing such explanations of its mode of action).

Although keen to explain the mechanism of acupuncture along the most 'modern' and 'scientific' lines, and thus to protect it from the tarnish of quackery, exponents of acupuncture were even more eager to spread the practice. They took to the rapidly expanding medical press, producing both case studies of its therapeutic successes and (even more copiously) experimental reports. Both types of account circulated widely, aided by the then-common practice in European and American medical journals of reprinting 'digests' of each other's more prominent articles. Perhaps even more effective in spreading information about the 'new' technique were the enthusiastic accounts of foreign medical students in Paris. Such first-hand descriptions of near-miraculous cures engaged personal as well as social networks, and helped to transmit the hands-on practice of acupuncture.

Investigations of the technique, particularly those driven by interest in electricity and its biological effects, spread across Europe. Trials took place in England, Scotland, Germany, France, Italy, the Low Countries, and the United States, as well as in more remote locations. Monographs, too, played an important role in propagating acupuncture. For example, the practice of acupuncture by the English-speaking profession was profoundly influenced by a single book: *A Treatise on Acupuncturation*, published by James Morss Churchill in 1822. Churchill's book, like Berlioz's text before it, introduced the healing needle through a disquisition on its 'Oriental' origins. Again like Berlioz, Churchill took pains to distinguish the practice of acupuncture in Europe from its practice in China, and to emphasize his own initial scepticism of Chinese claims for the technique:

I should not have taken the tales which are told of the wonderful cures effected by this operation amongst the original founders of it, as sufficient authority for recommending it, nor would I admit the fables which are promulgated by these people, as evidence of its efficacy, had not this efficacy been witnessed by European spectators on its native soil, and at length experienced in our own hemisphere; and even latterly, in our own country.[17]

Although he later gently chided his medical predecessors for their reluctance to adopt or even thoroughly test acupuncture, Churchill (unlike Busschof, who had made a similar complaint in relation to moxa) initially blamed that too on the Chinese themselves: 'It is probable, that the hyperbole in which it has been related, has induced the sober minds of our Northern soil, to treat these relations as the fictions of the Eastern imagination, and to reject them without examination, as fables.'[18] So that 'gay luxurious imagination' crops up again, but this time clearly marked as a liability, rather than a lesser virtue.

Fictional or not, by the second decade of the nineteenth century, the British, French, and American medical presses had succumbed to the forces of curiosity and rising interest, and began to report on acupuncture. For twenty years, studies of acupuncture, and cases of its success (and later of its failure) peppered medical periodicals. Physicians and surgeons in private and hospital practice alike experimented with the technique, and speculated on the cause of its curious effects. As the US-based commentator Dunglison noted in a compendium of 'new remedies' of the 1840s, '[a]lthough acupuncturation is really an ancient therapeutical agent, attention to it has been so much revived of late years, and its use has been so largely extended, that it may be looked upon as constituting one of the novelties of therapeutics':

M. Jules Cloquet had much to do with reviving its employment in his own country and elsewhere, by his treatise on the subject published at Paris, in 1826, where it was for a long period a fashionable article in the hospitals; so much so, it is affirmed, that attempts were even made to heal a fractured bone by it without the application of any appropriate apparatus! and at one time, it is said, the patients in one of the hospitals actually revolted against the *piqueurs médecins*.[19]

Laymen and -women too played a crucial role in increasing awareness of the technique and promoting its use by medical professionals. Patients were amazed by acupuncture's efficiency in relieving pain that had, in many cases, plagued them for years. Mr A. W., 'a corpulent man' afflicted with lumbago (lower back pain and stiffness, such as that caused muscle strain or a slipped disc), was reported by his Fulham surgeon as 'expressing the greatest astonishment at what he termed the "magical effect of the needles"!!!' The same surgeon reported of another patient, a poor woman with 'six infant children' (and thus, unsurprisingly, a bad back):

Although perfectly freed from pain, it was enough to excite a smile to witness the woman's scepticism on the success of the operation; she could scarcely credit her senses, for when desired to turn on her back she obeyed with hesitation, and doubt, dreading lest she should encounter the 'pain'. . . . It was very gratifying to see the poor creature sit up; her countenance beamed with delight, equalled only by her astonishment and grateful thanks for the 'wonderful cure' I wrought her.[20]

Another patient, this time Churchill's own, wrote an account of his illness and cure, at his doctor's request. Sick with pain and weakness in his left hip, unable to walk any distance, and generally debilitated by 'a residence in a tropical climate, together with indulging too freely in excesses, which destroyed the digestive powers', C. Lindo of Margate sought Churchill's opinion on his case. Churchill regarded it as unsuitable for acupuncture, and Lindo instead 'visited the whole round of celebrated regulars, and irregulars', without success. 'As a forlorn hope, and at his earnest desire', Churchill agreed to try out the needles. Lindo concluded his account: 'I derived temporary relief from acupuncture, there is not the least doubt, and had I at the time, the advantage of country air, it is probable that a more beneficial result might have accrued . . . '.[21] No miracle cure here, then, but after Lindo's unavailing round of treatments—including apparently, a caustic chemical rub that blistered him badly—his willingness to publicize a nearly painless, and at least temporarily beneficial, remedy is hardly surprising. Indeed one of the features most marked and discussed about acupuncture was that 'It would seem, that the operation is, as a general rule, most successful when it occasions the least pain.'[22] The consumer appeal of this unusual attribute can be readily imagined . . .

As had been the case for moxabustion (and as would be the case for homeopathy), socially prominent individuals played a crucial role in raising the visibility of acupuncture. In Britain, for example, one noble gout-sufferer—George O'Brien, Third Earl of Egremont, a noted patron of the racing world and member of the Prince-Regent's high-flying Brighton set—was cured of an excruciating, five-week bout of sciatica by acupuncture. In his relief, he paid the innovative surgeon a small fortune, renamed his favourite racehorse 'Acupuncture', and promoted the technique enthusiastically amongst his high-flying circle. As his well-rewarded surgeon recalled, 'There are no bounds to his Lordship's gratitude and delight: he went . . . to Brighton, a distance of thirty miles, to make it known amongst the nobility and faculty there.'[23] As with moxa in the eighteenth century, it was the existence of and interactions between lay and professional networks—local, national, and international—that facilitated the spread of acupuncture in the early and middle nineteenth century.

Another version of the Earl of Egremont's miraculous cure, told post-prandially in the clubrooms of a London medical society some five years later, offers additional evidence of acupuncture's specific attractions for both patients and medical professionals. A surgeon named Dendy recounted the tale with some considerable gusto. Rich in detail, his version differed from earlier accounts in several ways: first, he told his medical audience much more about the Earl's case—and especially about its intractability to orthodox cures. George O'Brien was clearly nothing if not determined; by the time he heard of acupuncture, he had endured every orthodox measure and several well-known quackish ones at the hands of 'every medical man of note in London'. They had availed him nothing: 'he retired to his seat at Petworth, in despair'. It was upon his arrival at Petworth that the central importance of both lay and professional networks in propagating acupuncture becomes evident.

A friend of mine [Martin], who resided in Sussex at that time, happened to get an early copy of Mr. Churchill's little work on acupuncture, and tried the remedy therein advocated with perfect success on an old woman who was a protégé of Lady Burrell, the daughter-in-law of the Earl. Her ladyship heard of the cure, and told the Earl what had been done; the result was, that the surgeon was sent for forthwith to try the new process on the peer.[24]

Martin, a surgeon, got his advanced copy because he and Churchill were acquainted in their student days at Guys and St Thomas's Hospitals. Sometimes, who you knew *determined* what you knew, and when. The Earl called Martin because of his daughter-in-law's network of charitable patronage. And O'Brien in turn deployed his own elite social network in acupuncture's cause.

But Dendy's enthusiasm waned as he came to the close of his tale. He admitted that he had himself no very good news to tell of the technique: 'When first it was proposed, it certainly effected some singular cures, but, of late, success does not seem to have attended it . . . As regards my own experience . . . I have lately had three cases in which I have tried this remedy without advantage.'[25] Neither Dendy nor his auditors offered any explanation of acupuncture's declining efficacy. Other contemporaries agued that the needle's early success had encouraged too many practitioners to use it as a panacea in unsuitable or indeed incurable cases. Certainly, by the 1840s, acupuncture was typically tried by doctors on precisely those patients whose ailments had proven particularly intransigent. No longer novel, nor sufficiently 'miraculous', acupuncture disappeared from the medical press almost as quickly as it had appeared.

The practice of acupuncture, however, continued. Dendy's story and the social setting within which it was told offer substantial clues to the mechanism of acupuncture's survival after its media heyday. Rarely in the spotlight of the medical periodicals, local groups like the London Medical Society offered a convivial space in which medical gentlemen could quietly exchange news and trade tips on the practice of medicine (as opposed to the often more contentious issues of theory). These societies were shaped both by traditions of gentlemanly amateurism and by the newer demands of competition and professionalization. In the nineteenth century, science and experiment remained largely the province of the amateur, and doctors were prominent participants in scientific and technical innovation and debate. Medical men pursued both as matters of interest and in pursuit of gains tangible and intangible. With increased training in the 'allied sciences' of medicine, doctors considered themselves uniquely well able to evaluate mesmerism, galvanism, new drugs, the use of the stethoscope, and myriad other medical innovations of indeterminate worth—including acupuncture—and gathered together to do so in precisely these settings. Thus, although periodicals were a crucial mechanism by which to propagate a new technique, they were far from the only one.

Churchill himself had initially learned of acupuncture not from reading the published French reports of it, but from another surgeon, Mr Scott of Westminster. Churchill's interest was aroused by privately communicated and subsequently directly witnessed successes with needling. Even before he published his *Treatise on Acupuncturation*, Churchill was part of a growing nexus of British practitioners interested in or using acupuncture. And he tapped into the power of such personal networks himself as he struggled both to popularize and to standardize acupuncture practice. Churchill actively sought out acupuncture success stories and collected cases in which his adopted technique had procured long-sought health. He was not alone in this endeavour; at least one prominent patient insisted that his doctors not only learn the technique (as propounded by Churchill), but that they report their successes back to him for further distribution. Another valuable tool for fostering acupuncture's credibility and inculcating its practice was eye-witnessing. Just as Churchill had been converted to acupuncture by seeing it in action, so others were brought into the fold. The act of witnessing was a frequent point of contact and potential transmission, and one that also illuminates (changing) contemporary structures of authority and its propagation. At the beginning of the century and for some considerable period, Churchill and his successors regularly listed the names of socially prominent observers who were in attendance upon successfully cured acupuncture patients, implying that their presence added weight to the reported results.[26] But this model of authority was in decline within medicine. By the mid-century, it was slowly being replaced by statistics and by large-scale clinical observation.

This proved a stumbling block for acupuncture's proponents. Most of the men who publicly supported acupuncture depended on their practices for both livelihood and 'clinical material' (patients). In a second volume, presenting case studies proving the efficacy of acupuncture, Churchill complained that he could not perform the experiments necessary to establish acupuncture's active principle because his small practice threw up insufficient numbers of appropriate cases.[27] This dilemma only worsened as the century progressed and the single case study lost its primacy in the periodical literature. Acupuncture supporters found themselves reporting on individual cases even after the multiple case study had become the norm for testing the efficacy of a medical practice or innovation. But what could they do? They often saw little chance of another suitable case appearing in their practices. Reporting late in the century on a solitary case in which acupuncture had relieved the pain of a man dying from cancer, one such practitioner prefaced his datum with the apologetic acknowledgement:

[O]ne case goes only a short way in establishing any method of alleviating or curing the pain of this formidable disease, but a long interval may pass before another presents itself in a small provincial town with a sparse surrounding population. Hence my reason for publishing a single case.[28]

As the balance in medicine tilted away from 'art' and toward 'science', the power of individual practitioners in private practice to significantly influence medical practice diminished. Often silent in the face of 'scientific medicine', such practitioners still had to satisfy their patients at the bedside, where doctors still struggled to establish themselves as the exclusive interpreters of the body. Day-to-day medicine remained a social art, and the laity, heterodox practitioners, midwives, and others still claimed the right to observe the body and pronounce upon it authoritatively. Patients demanded particular cures based on what they saw, and acupuncture's near-invisibility in the medical press limited lay awareness of the technique as well. Acupuncture's proponents may have regarded a blandly empirical westernization as more readily assimilable, but it was hardly attention-grabbing. Certainly it lacked in drama, particularly as adversarial new systems like homeopathy emerged to offer formidable competition to merely orthodox alternatives, and controversy swept the medical and popular presses.

As an explicitly and vocally alternative medical system originating in a European context, homeopathy offers an excellent foil to acupuncture's non-European origins, and to its status as an apparently unthreatening stand-alone innovation. Moreover, where the history of acupuncture in Europe is cyclic and discontinuous, the history of homeopathy is continuous, illuminating the impact of changes in the institutions of biomedicine on medical systems which opposed it. So what can the history of homeopathy in the nineteenth century tell us about nineteenth-century responses to acupuncture?

The Local Opposition: Homeopathy and 'Alternative' Medicine

First, it may be worthwhile to spell out the similarities between homeopathy and acupuncture as each emerged from the marketplace pluralism of the eighteenth century into the medical monopoly-building of the nineteenth. As I've described, both homeopathy and acupuncture depended heavily—at least in theory—on subjective accounts of sensation and experience. Homeopathic doctors used their own experiences and sensations to 'prove' drugs. Homeopathic diagnosis relied heavily on patient self-reporting, and on the equally subjective accounts of the patient's friends and family. And certainly the mechanism by which homeopathic medicines produced their effects was mysterious: how could medicines composed almost entirely of water produce *any* effect on the sick body, much less a curative one? Neither was initially conceived as an 'alternative' in the sense in which we use the term today—as an either/or proposition. Acupuncture's proponents (like the advocates of mesmerism) wished to add new weapons to orthodoxy's armoury in the battle against disease, while homeopaths expected their system to gradually displace by expansion the inferior techniques of allopathy, while absorbing its useful accumulated knowledge.

However, like orthodox medicine—or, as homeopathists rather polemically described it, 'allopathy'—homeopathy was, and was understood to be, a fully elaborated system of medical thought. In other words, both lay and professional responses to homeopathy took into account its theory and its practices as well as its material culture (the drugs themselves). Moreover, as we saw, over the course of the nineteenth century homeopathists developed their own professional journals, medical societies, research institutes, hospitals, medical schools, and even corporate pharmaceutical offshoots. Reactions to homeopathy from within the orthodox profession, although initially moderate and assimilative, rapidly became violently hostile (if still, surreptitiously, assimilative). And this hostility had a profound effect: rules like those of the AMA and BMA forbidding any consultation or cooperation between their members and 'homeopathists' and mandating the expulsion of any member caught 'dabbling' with homeopathy forced a unitary identity upon the wide range of healers who took up the system. Whatever their training, whatever the degree of their belief in Hahnemann's principles, all were equally 'homeopathists' in the eyes of their professional organizations. No such judgements or demands were made of regulars who chose to use acupuncture; one could easily take up the needle without taking up the title 'acupuncturist'—and indeed few if any even of acupuncture's most eloquent proponents would have defined themselves in terms of their use of the technique. Each of these differences played a crucial role in acupuncture's failure to thrive, or to challenge established medical models in the way that homeopathy did so successfully.

To render acupuncture assimilable by the 'regular' medical profession at the beginning of the nineteenth century, its proponents
had relied on the pragmatism of the average practitioner and
patient, and presented it as simply, empirically, an effective treatment for particular ailments. And at the beginning of the nineteenth
century, good empirical evidence of success in particular cases was
enough; a culturally challenging theory for which no material
evidence could be found was considerably worse than no theory
at all, at least in terms of rendering acupuncture acceptable. After
the mid-century, however, this was no longer the case; pure
empiricism (particularly when disconnected from even the possibility
of a material explanation) was becoming a threat to the profession's
aspirations to scientificity and the social authority that came with
it. Empiricism was slipping back into the hands of the 'quacks'. But
by then, western practitioners of acupuncture had become so habitu-
ated to trial-by-error needling *in locus dolenti* that its lost theoretical
basis would in any case have been almost irrelevant.

By the same token, acupuncture users, lacking a unitary identity—
they were consultant surgeons and physicians, general practitioners,
and very occasionally late in the century also followers of the new
'specialities' such as neurology—and not excluded from the orthodox
medical communion, felt no impulse to create their own institutions. In particular, they created no centres of training; individuals
like Elliotson might mention acupuncture in lectures, or demonstrate it on teaching rounds should a suitable case be present. As
long as acupuncture remained novel (and as long as its prominent
practitioners remained orthodox!) such mentions could gain wide
audiences: both lectures and notes on ward rounds were often
serialized by the medical periodicals. But as acupuncture became
familiar, its use—limited as it was to relatively minor and unexciting
ailments—was no longer worthy of mention. Such essentially op-
portunistic efforts could not substitute for inclusion in a formal
education programme, once the medical press turned its spotlight
elsewhere. On the other hand, local cultures of acupuncture use
persisted; for instance, it was 'for years a favourite traditional practice at the Leeds Infirmary' where three generations of Pridgin

Teales used it as Surgeons to the Infirmary.[29] But informal networks and family traditions were increasingly peripheral to the process by which innovations in medicine were diffused and entered the mainstream. Periodicals, textbooks, and formal medical education had, by the end of the nineteenth century, become the essential media for the transmission of medical knowledge. Homeopaths, precisely because of their formal exclusion from these venues, were well prepared for this shift, with journals, schools, and textbooks of their own, through which to propagate succeeding generations of homeopathic practitioners.

In fact, the case of homeopathy usefully illustrates both the benefits and the disadvantages of the 'alternative' position/posture. Clearly, homeopathists and supporters of homeopathy used the rhetoric of opposition to—and oppression by—medical orthodoxy to draw attention to the flaws of allopathic practice and the distinctiveness of their own. This in turn allowed them to build a strong and visible identity, which could be shared by professionals, amateurs, and consumers alike. However, by choosing to position homeopathy as an alternative to orthodox medicine, and by defining their therapy in part by what it was not, homeopathy's proponents left homeopathy open to being grouped with all the other self-proclaimed 'alternatives', ranging from the medically respectable (such as osteopathy) to the downright disreputable (clairvoyance, for example). Similarly, by promoting homeopathy as an exclusive choice, they brought upon themselves the same set of disadvantages that faced allopaths in their battles to exclude homeopathy. The adversarial approach also encouraged dogmatism among homeopathic 'purists', which in turn reduced the flexibility of modernizers to incorporate popular new techniques or respond to challenging new doctrines, like germ theory. If acupuncture was rendered amorphous in the absence of theory, homeopathy was rendered brittle by an overly rigid theoretical structure.

And that brings us again to the question of culture, and the cross-cultural specificity (or not) of medicine. Were the different responses to and trajectories of acupuncture and homeopathy influenced by the fact that the former originated in China and the latter in Europe, and if so in what ways? Certainly, the separation of practice from theory in the case of acupuncture was intimately related to European perceptions of Chinese natural and medical knowledge as devoid of merit (beyond its antiquarian interest as an earlier stage of civilization). Those perceptions, as Floyer's diligent efforts of translation suggest, related not just to the factual content of that body of knowledge (on what side of the body the heart was lodged; the length of the intestines; the rate of circulation in the body) but to the cosmologies and epistemologies embedded therein (a non-dichotomous universe, a body internally legible through physical sensations, rather than auditory clues or direct inspection) and the manner in which the substance of each of these categories was expressed ('flowery', 'poetical' language). But perceptions of cross-cultural medical expertise were also influenced by far less arcane matters: for instance, the politics of international trade. Simply put, when Britain's political and economic relationship with China was, or was expected to be profitable, British attitudes towards China and all things Chinese tended to be buoyant. When that relationship soured, as it did after the failure of successive missions to China seeking more favourable trading terms, and in the period preceding and during the Opium Wars, so did attitudes towards other aspects of Chinese culture.

In the 1820s, when Churchill was first promoting the use of acupuncture in Britain, Lord Amherst had recently returned from a British ambassadorial mission to China in the years 1816 and 1817. The end of the Napoleonic Wars had allowed the re-expansion of British diplomatic and economic horizons, and the rigidity of the Canton Cohong system was again a focus for anti-Chinese sentiments. Moreover, the Country (private) traders were simultaneously pressing for the ending of the East India Company's monopoly of the China trade, and illicitly expanding their own ventures in East Asia. The embassy was ignominiously expelled from China without even a formal audience with the Emperor, much less any new agreement on trade terms. The embarrassing failure of Amherst's mission contributed to growing (elite) British disgust with China in general and the Chinese government in particular. In the popular press, the British public read tales of Chinese medicine and technology, set in the context of an obstinate and autocratic government. Perhaps even worse, at least for perceptions of Chinese medicine, they were told that Britain's generous attempt to negotiate had been blocked by a Chinese doctor.

China during this period gallingly persisted in regarding itself as self-sufficient, and culturally superior. Consequently, it did not seek to ally itself with or learn from European nations, and regarded its many foreign visitors and inhabitants as mere pilgrims to the shrine of a higher culture. Embassies from European powers were routinely referred to as 'tribute envoys' and required to follow long-established schedules, routes, and rituals. The Amherst mission evaded these rules (arguing that it was not a tribute mission) and attempted to establish its own pace and precedents—or as the Chinese officials perceived it, stalled and prevaricated. On the Embassy's arrival in Beijing, Amherst was immediately summoned to the Emperor's presence. He declined, on the grounds of illness, and begged for time to recover. The Emperor immediately offered the assistance of his own physician:

The Ambassador was immediately visited by the promised physician. This gentleman, who appeared to be something beyond the middle age, was dressed as a Mandarin. He felt His Lordship's pulse in both wrists; and having observed that his stomach was probably disordered from the use of a Chinese diet, recommended repose and an emetic, and retired. The report of this person to the Emperor, materially influenced, as it afterwards appeared, our subsequent treatment.

In other words, the imperial physician appears to have reported that Amherst was faking illness; as this was apparently the only reason given to the Emperor for the Ambassador's refusal to attend him, the Embassy was disgraced.[30] Unsurprisingly, a considerable number of pages and column inches reporting and discussing the failed mission were expended on critiques of Chinese medical knowledge and theory, and the 'absurdities' of its practices. In particular, Chinese practitioners were criticized as 'entirely destitute of anatomical knowledge'.[31] As the *Lancet* scoffed,

The knowledge of Anatomy among these primitive people is extremely slight and superficial. . . . The existence of the great viscera of the chest and abdomen is certainly ascertained, but the Chinese are profoundly ignorant of their relative position. The heart is thus supposed by them to be on the right side and the liver on the left.—There is scarcely an allusion made to the nervous, fibrous, and muscular structures. . . . In Physiology the Chinese are seen to scarcely less disadvantage.[32]

At first glance, this hostility seems to have had little effect on perceptions of acupuncture—after all, it was in the first flush of its British glory in the 1820s and 1830s—but of course, it does explain the urgency with which Churchill and other acupuncture supporters worked to cut acupuncture's ties with China, and to define their practice of acupuncture as anatomically based. Moreover, particularly in medical forums, they presented France, rather than China, as the immediate origin of European acupuncture, both in terms of its intellectual and its empirical antecedents. Obviously, Churchill and his counterparts knew that acupuncture was developed in China, but few traces of China persisted in the description and practice of acupuncture in Britain in the face of that nation's growing unpopularity. Even the needles themselves were domesticated and, westernized—this not only stripped them of undesirably 'Chinese' attributes, but powerfully illustrated the ease with which practitioners could construct their own apparatus to test the new treatment (see Figure 17).

Contemporary observers were certainly aware of a close relationship between popular attitudes towards different cultures and public medical enthusiasms. Britain's victory over China in the Opium Wars enabled Britain to negotiate her own trade terms, punitive damages, and perhaps most importantly, healed British *amour-propre*, wounded by Chinese indifference to British trade and British culture. In its wake, orthodox medical practitioners contemplated the likely effects of increased exchange with the Chinese.[33] Some even saw stirrings of a medical equivalent to the eighteenth-century chinoiserie craze, which had itself occurred during a period of greater openness in the China trade and correspondingly positive perceptions of China. In 1844, a scandalized but anonymous 'Medical Practitioner' scolded the government for its lax attitudes towards quacks in general, from mesmerists to dentists (for specialism—the notion that one could understand and treat one

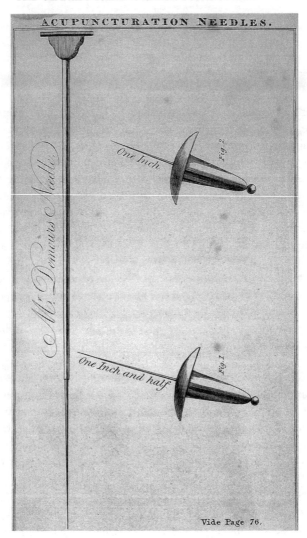

17. 'Mr Demour's needle', from James Morss Churchill, *A Treatise on Acupuncturation*, 1821. Still a simple technology, the acupuncture needle here is a very western one, designed to ease the fears of European and North American patients uncomfortable with the idea of needling and fearful that the needle might become lost in the body. Compare with the exotic needle of Figure 13.

part of the human organism in isolation from its systemic context—
was itself seen as a sort of quackery until the late nineteenth century).
In the midst of his tirade, the author singled out 'for its bare-faced
impudence' the 'Chinese pills', as exemplifying all the frauds from
which the Government should be protecting its citizens:

No sooner had the news of peace having been made in China reached us,
then a 'most important discovery' was announced, and 'Chinese Pills' were
placarded throughout the kingdom, recommended as a 'Universal remedy,' their virtues transcendently soaring above those of all other universal
remedies hitherto known... What, I ask, is the humble, unlettered,
labouring man to think of these lies about the Chinese Physician's effectual
means for contending with disease? He knows not but that all there stated
may be true; he knows not that the Chinese theory and practice of
Medicine is about as correct, in most of its principles, as the vain conceit
of their own celestial relationship; that it is, in fact, the deepest in the dark,
of all the intellectual pursuits of that singular people.[34]

Other authors were less perturbed, but nonetheless recognized that
the forced opening of China was likely to bring new competitors to
the medical scene. John Wilson, Medical Inspector of Naval Hospitals and Fleets, and recently returned from duty in China, mused
in 1844: 'There is no saying whether, among the curiosities which
will find their way hence to London, a celestial doctor may not be
one.' Perhaps Wilson's complacency stemmed from his quite accurate view that Chinese medicine would compete far more directly with homeopathy than with orthodoxy:

He [the hypothetical Chinese practitioner] would possess pre-eminently
the charm of novelty; and if to that he added the irresistible recommendation of boasting loudly, and boldly professing his power to cure all
manner of disease, he might prove a formidable rival to the homeopathist.
At any rate, he would be his fit antagonist, and a pretty race might be run
between them for the popular favour. It is suspected, however, that the
expounder of the pun-tsaow would be beaten, principally though
the burthen of his big boluses, by the light weight of the disciple of
Hahnemann; for the imaginative invalid who delights to toy with the
immeasurable minute doses of the latter, would be frightened or disgusted
by the drenches and balls of the former.[35]

In the end, if a 'celestial doctor' came to Britain in the decades after the Opium Wars, he or she left no traces on British medical culture. 'Chinese pills' and similar Orientalized patent medicines came and went. Acupuncture remained, albeit in its highly westernized form, embedded in local cultures and private practices. Its proponents occasionally grabbed the spotlight of the medical periodicals with unusual case studies, and more rarely, clinical studies in hospitals. One 'quack' practice associated itself with acupuncture: Baunscheidtism, used most famously to treat male sexual dysfunction and involving the use of a spring-loaded array of blades or needles and an irritating ointment applied to the site of puncture to create an eruptive rash. But in general, the practice of therapeutic needling stayed free from such taints, and firmly within (although peripheral to) orthodox practice across Europe and North America until the closing years of the nineteenth century.

As I and other historians have argued, the rise of homeopathy ended the reign of 'heroic medicine' and promoted the growth of a unified (and monopolistic) orthodox medical profession (see Chapter 2). Acupuncture certainly had no such profound effects, although arguably its advent and popularity did help to familiarize and domesticate the needle itself as a medical instrument. By the end of the nineteenth century, needles were commonly used to treat aneurism, to relieve various forms of edema, to introduce vaccine matter, and the hypodermic needle and syringe was being introduced; proponents of each of these innovations all harked back to acupuncture's relative safety and painlessness as evidence that they too were safe. In the first decades of the twentieth century, changes in medical education and in the structures of medical practice, and the rise of new therapies for the treatment of ailments like tetanus, rheumatism, neuralgia, gout, and sciatica—and perhaps most importantly, a rising sense amongst the orthodox medical profession of the power of the new scientific medicine—saw acupuncture drop out of western practice altogether. It would not return to its early nineteenth-century heights of popularity until the 1960s and 1970s.

4

'WITH OUR WESTERN BRETHREN, THE CASE SEEMS TO BE QUITE DIFFERENT'

The preceding chapters have looked at and compared interactions between medical systems—western and non-western, orthodox and heterodox—as they transpired in the West, where a single, increasingly dominant medical system has long sought an absolute monopoly over healing practices and theories. But what happens when medical systems come into contact in a setting which is already highly pluralistic, and where no single system has achieved even a nominal dominance, or where monopoly is not posited as the ultimate goal of medical system? Can there be 'alternative medicine' in the absence of medical monopolism? And are the cultural, social, political, and material factors that influence the medical marketplace and shape the choices and strategies of medical consumers significantly different when pluralism is the accepted norm? To explore these aspects of cross-cultural and alternative medicine, we must look beyond Europe and North America.[1]

By studying responses to cross-cultural medical expertise in the West, I have inevitably also been studying western attitudes towards the non-western world. But of course, western medical systems have themselves been exported. In fact, western medicine was, from at least the nineteenth century (and is still today) widely regarded as the most effective and indeed humane 'tool of empire'. As the *Indian Medical Gazette* (quasi-official mouthpiece of the Indian Medical Service and thus of the largest body of western medical men active in imperial India) editorialized in 1887: 'Ever since the arrival of the English in

India, the services of medical officers have been recognized by the military and civil authorities as extremely valuable in rendering the yoke of foreign domination more easy to be tolerated by the people, and in popularizing English rule.'[2] Western doctors working in the non-western world spoke often of 'medical missions' and missionaries, and regarded their medical work as serving not merely sick individuals but also sick and decaying civilizations—views which naturally coloured their perceptions of the medical expertise produced by those cultures. Thus to better understand the phenomena of cross-cultural and alternative medicine in a global context, we must see it also from a slightly different angle: from within colonized, as well as colonizing, cultures. This chapter interrogates responses to novel medical practices and systems in India.

Medicine beyond the Monoculture: India and Medical Pluralism

Although there were individuals, and in Goa communities, from Europe in India from at least the sixteenth century, their influence was limited, and their medical practitioners competed—both intellectually and commercially—with their indigenous counterparts on a more or less equal footing. European doctors were certainly given prerogatives within European settlements, but Indian practitioners of various systems were often similarly privileged by their own communities. Some lay members of all communities actively sought treatment from doctors of other schools, and some practitioners from each community were equally active in seeking to exchange medical knowledge. European doctors were well aware that their own medical expertise was shaped by northern climes. Given the established model of the humoural body as existing in dynamic equilibrium with the environment, they knew that their familiar cures and practices might well prove ill-suited to the very different conditions of the tropics. The marked tendency for transplanted Europeans to sicken and die in hot climates merely confirmed this view. As one English physician practising in India in the late seventeenth century put it, 'We are here, as Exotick Plants brought home to us, not agreeable to the Soil.'[3] Thus they were often eager to tap into local medical knowledge. A Jesuit narrator described the synergy he had seen on the ground in Portuguese Goa (and incidentally demonstrated the persistence of close connections between medicine and religion in Europe in this period):

I knew a friar of St. Augustine, of the Portuguese nation, who taught medicine in Portugal, and lectured on it for 16 years, who after coming to India treated some Portuguese patients, all of who passed away; seeing this happening, the said priest called the Panditas and asked them how they went about curing their patients; they replied that the properties and compositions of the drugs were well taught in the books; however, this was not sufficient to heal the patient unless his complexion, and the ruling humour, and the connection with the local climate were first known, and that they ordered their remedies according to these principles. Knowing they were giving him a good reason, the Priest took some information from them in order to succeed in curing, and according to this and his science, he later made some wonderful cures.[4]

Two things really stand out in this passage: first, it illustrates the similarities between and basic compatibility of European and Indian medical theory in this period. Second, it hints at the trends that would, as we saw in Chapters 1 and 3, divide them: our medical friar was willing and able to learn from his local counterparts, but his subsequent 'wonderful cures' were rooted, in his own eyes and those of his European contemporaries not in sedulously following indigenous practices, but in combining them with 'his science'.

Europeans had another very good reason to cultivate medical contacts amongst local experts: they were often desperately short of familiar medicaments, many of which had to be shipped expensively from Europe. Even those items in the European pharmacopoeia which originated in Asia were often tantalizingly out of reach—because of course they were known and sold in India not by their European but by their local names, and might appear in different forms in the marketplace. Moreover, the providential notion that a benevolent divinity had placed in any locale the appropriate remedies for its particular prevailing ills endured into the nineteenth century, and encouraged doctors to seek local cures for local diseases. So one prominent aspect of the cross-cultural encounter—and by far the most durable one, persisting as it does today—was a mining of indigenous pharmacopoeia by foreign medical practitioners, and the corporate and governmental entities they served. Again and again, bureaucratic authorities and enthusiastic amateurs alike exhorted medical men on the ground to systematically collect information about local drugs and medical botanicals. In 1784, the Asiatic Society (later, the Asiatic Society of Bengal) was founded in India; in his inaugural address, its first president Sir William Jones issued its members a broad remit:

You will investigate whatever is rare in the stupendous fabrick of nature; will correct the geography of Asia by new observations and discoveries; will trace the annals, and even traditions, of those nations who, from time to time, have peopled or desolated it; and will bring to light their various institutions civil and religious. You will examine their improvements and methods in arithmetick and geometry, in trigonometry, mensuration, mechanicks, opticks, astronomy, and general physicks; their systems of morality, grammar, rhetorick and dialectick; their skill in chirurgery and medicine; and their advancement, whatever it may be, in anatomy and chemistry. To this you will add researches into their agriculture, manufactures, trade; and while you inquire with pleasure into their musick, architecture, painting and poetry, will not neglect those inferior arts by which the comforts, and even elegancies, of social life are supplied and improved.[5]

In fact, Jones cited Engelbert Kaempfer (see Chapter 2) as a model for such inquiries, and suggested that 'native' authors too be published in the papers of the Society. A year later, however, his address focused much more tightly on medicine—and on indigenous plant medicines and local decoctions. These he portrayed as far more valuable than complex drugs or classical texts, however 'judicious and rational' earlier generations of European medics had found them:

So highly has medical skill been prized by the ancient *Indians*, that one of the *fourteen Retna's*, or *precious things*, which the gods produced by churning the ocean with the mountain *Mandara*, was a *learned physician*. What their old books contain on this subject we ought certainly to discover . . . but we can expect nothing so important from the works of *Hindu* and *Muselman* physicians, as the knowledge which experience must have given them, of simple medicines. I have seen an *Indian* prescription of *fifty-four*, and another of *fifty-six*, ingredients; but such compositions are always to be suspected . . . and it were better to find certain accounts of a single leaf or berry, than to be acquainted with the most elaborate compounds, unless they too have been proved by a multitude of successful experiments.[6]

The process of extracting such knowledge was neither straightforward nor simple. Francis Buchanan, medical officer on the Syme mission to Burma in 1796–8, recorded in his journal what must have been a fairly typical encounter:

June 16. This morning I visited the Burma Doctor he had a good house with a number of good looking women about it and a large garden. He had a number of plants both in his garden and in large baskets in his house among others . . . one of them a fine amonium was in flower, but although he dug up a large bulbous root of it I could not persuade him to let me take a scapus [a plant of the lily family] in flower in order to be able to examine it.

As Buchanan's grumblings illustrate, westerners were far from in control of these meetings; the exchange had to be negotiated and, like it or not, western medical prospectors were very much dependent on the goodwill of indigenous experts. But Buchanan was to be further tried: 'I was much vexed and more so by being obliged to hear a long story from him which I could not understand concerning the virtues of each plant. One was good for the blood (Boerhavia diffusa), another for the wind, one was hot, another cold, and one . . . was good for everything.'[7] His clear frustration is very revealing: not only was his interlocutor taking up his time with, to him, incomprehensible exegesis, but even the parts of his account which Buchanan could understand sounded of dubious value to his western ears.

As European medicine became increasingly materialistic, the kinds of information its travelling representatives sought changed. Whereas very early accounts often included descriptions of traditions surrounding the compounding, prescription, and application of different medical substances (Kaempfer, for example, offered a detailed description of the astrologically timed harvesting and preparation of the moxa fibres), later doctors reported on the

materia medica alone, or detailed associated 'native' medical practices merely for their antiquarian interest. The 1830s, for example,
saw the Calcutta Medical and Physical Society form a 'Committee
of Inquiry upon the Vegetable, Animal and Mineral Productions of
Medicinal Qualities Procurable in India and the Surrounding
Countries'. This Committee posed a detailed set of questions to
its members, officers of the Indian Medical Service, and other
western medics working in the country. Their aim was to gather
a comprehensive inventory of available drugs in use among western
doctors and surgeons across the subcontinent.

What are the medicinal plants grown in the vicinity already, and the
measures which might be taken for extending the cultivation of them? . . .
What are the medical and chemical preparations made in the district from
vegetables used in medicine? . . . What are the mines and other localities
yielding crude mineral substances, and the quantities of them attainable for
medical purposes? . . . What are the preparations of these now manufactured,
and the practicability of producing them on a more extensive scale?[8]

Further questions attempted to ascertain what was available in area
markets, at what prices, and—almost as an afterthought—how local
healers used such substances.

But expropriation of natural knowledge and medical expertise
was far from unidirectional; from the sixteenth century on, Indians
had themselves been actively drawing on the recognized strength of
European medicine in surgery. Similarly, as soon as it became
affordable, medical practitioners across South Asia adopted the use
of the cinchona bark which had initially been brought by Europeans from the New World to their tropical trading posts and
settlements to treat malaria and other fevers.

Cross-cultural medical exchanges were not always voluntary or
driven by market forces. By the 1760s, after British forces had
defeated the French, the British began to consolidate and system-
atize their hold on the subcontinent. Many more Britons travelled
and settled in India as soldiers, traders, bureaucrats, teachers, and
missionaries—and with them came their doctors, their medical
traditions, and an overwhelming sense of the superiority of their

culture. This sometimes overbearing cultural self-confidence combined with the forces of military and economic consolidation in the form of the 'civilizing mission'. And as I've suggested above, medicine was to play a central role in that mission.

The British response to smallpox in India offers one of the clearest and earliest examples of the fit between medicine and the 'civilizing mission'. Before the nineteenth century, smallpox was one of relatively few diseases recognized by westerners and non-westerners alike as 'specific' and contagious: as being a distinctive entity whose form was stable and essentially predictable in every affected individual, rather than an idiosyncratic imbalance of humours and environment. It was also one of very few serious diseases that could be regarded as in any way preventable: Asians had long used the technique of variolation (controlled exposure to a carefully selected mild case of smallpox) to produce immunity to the disease.[9] The technique had been transmitted to Europe through the efforts of (among others) Mary Wortley Montagu, wife of the British Ambassador to Turkey in the early eighteenth century. Variolation was by no means a certain method of producing the lifelong immunity conferred by surviving smallpox, nor was it an entirely safe one; Britons were, in fact, quite slow to accept it. But the disease in its natural form was so deadly, and so devastating even to its survivors that the risks of variolation were often acceptable to both individuals and communities. And this was the common, rather precarious position of Europe and India until the late eighteenth century, when Edward Jenner made his famous realization that individuals who survived the very mild cowpox were also immune to smallpox. Based on this discovery (or more accurately, this revelation to the medical elite of knowledge long held by the laypeople most affected), Jenner devised new method of preventing smallpox: vaccination (from 'vacca', or cow) with cowpox serum. Vaccination was vastly safer; it was also, at least in northern Europe where cowpox was endemic and vaccines could be fresh, more reliable and convenient. And it did not put communities at risk, as did ill-advised or sloppily practised variolation—with its consequent exposure of a community to virulent smallpox. The British regarded vaccination as a great gift

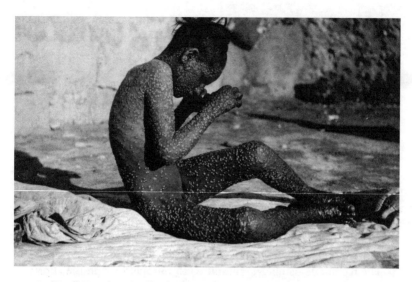

18. 'Small Pox [acquired] 9th day in Hospital', photograph from an early twentieth-century album, depicting a young Palestinian boy ravaged by small-pox in 1922.

that western medicine could bring to the colonial world—and a spectacular tool for persuading that world both of the superiority of European culture, and of the humanitarian virtues and practical benefits of empire. It was enthusiastically embraced by the Honourable East India Company (then administering India); one Company Agent described it as offering 'an additional mark of the fostering care of the British Government'. As early as 1803, when vaccination was first introduced in Bombay, the governor of the province expressed his confident belief that 'the prestige that we have achieved by this one act has been the source of much good will from the people—it is a great reward.'[10]

But if they expected vaccination to smooth the path of empire, or even to enhance the status and increase the popularity of western medicine, British officials and bureaucrats were doomed to disappointment. Vaccination, whatever its virtues and efficacy in Europe, met with considerable opposition, and experienced significant technical difficulties in India. And the British, who had expected gratitude and praise for their not inconsiderable investment in spreading what they saw as a clearly superior practice, were furious. Many looked to superstition, ignorance, fear of change, and religious dogmatism as explanation of Indian intransigence, ignoring the unreliability of early vaccines and abuses in their delivery (and indeed the fierce opposition faced by vaccination in Britain itself). They also blamed traditional practices and practitioners for the continued prevalence of smallpox, and tried to suppress variolation, while making vaccination compulsory, at least in certain areas and lines of work—those in which Indians were most likely to interact with Europeans. British authorities never doubted the virtues of vaccination, nor its suitability to India—nor, indeed, their own benevolence in introducing and mandating the practice. Cultural compromises, technical improvements, support from elite Indians, and experience gradually eroded public resistance to vaccination, but smallpox was not eliminated from India until 1975, well after decolonization had terminated British interventions, and broken the link between vaccination and empire.

Other diseases, too, came under the scrutiny—if not wholly under the control—of the Raj. The plague and cholera in particular offered opportunities for the Indian bureaucracy to leaven political and economic imperatives with a strong dose of medical justification and encouragement to assimilation, modernization, and westernization. Cholera and plague shared two important aspects: first, their epidemic spread threatened the economics of empire; second, their control seemed to demand major, expensive, and culturally disruptive social and sanitary interventions. In the face of repeated outbreaks in West of both diseases, Britain was faced with the unappealing prospect of either imposing quarantine or enduring embargoes of its Indian ports and shipping. These threats, as well as the horrific loss of life caused by the two diseases, stirred the Raj into public health action. Rendered less blithely confident of gratitude by the vaccination episode, and more cautious by the uprising of 1857, the Government of India tackled cholera at the mid-century with some reluctance, and only in the face of the intense international pressure. At the 1866 International Sanitary Conference at Constantinople, Britain was pointedly reminded of its special responsibility to fight cholera, based on its stewardship of India and its 'armies' of contagious pilgrims, then seen as 'the most powerful of all causes which conduce to the development and to the propagation of epidemics of cholera.'[11] A subsequent essayist spelled it out even more clearly: 'The squalid pilgrim army . . . with its rags and hair and skin freighted with vermin and impregnated with infection, may any year slay thousands of the most talented and beautiful of our age in Vienna, London, or Washington.'[12] The rather obvious fact that few Indian pilgrims had Vienna, London, or Washington in their travel plans—and that pilgrims were therefore unlikely to be direct vectors for cholera in Europe—was politely ignored by all: pilgrimage was much disliked and distrusted by British authorities in India; the religions of India in general, and particularly Hinduism, were widely regarded as degraded and distasteful. Changing or constraining such unacceptable practices was an attractive option, particularly if a neutral or humanitarian justification was available—like the need to protect the populations of India and the West from cholera. But the Government of India faced three serious deterrents. First, the proclamation of religious toleration issued by Queen Victoria in 1858, in the wake of the 'Mutiny', militated against any moves to block pilgrimage: 'The spread of cholera is no doubt a great evil but the awakening of a feeling of mistrust throughout India would be a greater evil still' argued Lord Roberts, who had experienced India in the grip of 'Mutiny' at first hand.[13] Second, neither doctors nor public health workers could agree on a single explanation for cholera—nor, therefore, on a plan to halt spread of the disease, or a cure for it. And finally, Britain had no wish to give additional force to contagionist calls for quarantines or other limits to the free movement of people or goods. The Government therefore acted slowly, hesitantly—and still faced outraged opposition from a wary Indian public, which had also not forgotten the 'Mutiny', or the problems with smallpox vaccinations.

Popular, medical, and administrative responses to the plague epidemics at the close of the nineteenth century illustrate the next phase of the interaction between medicine and empire. Unlike cholera, with its mysterious and much-contested aetiology, the western medical community in India rapidly reached a consensus that plague was contagious, caused by a micro-organism, and therefore that its dangers were embedded in and spread by the individual sick body. In part this was because the disease first struck on a massive scale in 1896, when germ theory was better established, at least in the medical community. This consensus, and the growing credibility of medical explanations and arguments in general, convinced Indian civil authorities to take medical advice far more seriously. Plague was also an urban disease in India, and therefore immediately threatening to domestic Indian manufacturing and business as well as international trade. Action was imperative— and it was draconian. Civil liberties and community standards were given short shrift; suspected Indian plague victims (Europeans were exempt) were forcibly examined, and if found to be infected, they were quarantined or hospitalized and their personal property destroyed. These actions violated caste practices, and infringed dearly held social and religious principles—especially where women were concerned. 'Native Ladies will prefer death to the humiliation of having their groins examined by male doctors who are utter strangers to them', one Indian newspaper proclaimed; another argued that the new plague laws permitted Indians to be treated like 'mere beasts and as such not entitled to any belief or sympathy'.[14] Even the bodies of the dead were not sacrosanct; they could be seized, dissected, and traditional funeral rites severely curtailed. Plague was also used by the Government to snatch back hard-won pockets of 'native agency'—to reduce the degree of self-governance attained in preceding decades by Indian cities, on the grounds that Indian-controlled municipal bodies were not acting strongly enough to control the epidemics. Unsurprisingly these astonishingly harsh and confrontational policies contained the seeds of their own demise. Indian civil unrest and protest rapidly reached alarming levels, while mass resistance to the measures rendered them ineffective. Colonial administrators realized that they would have to use persuasion and education, rather than direct coercion, however medically justified. In part because of such conciliatory and educational approaches, even during the plague epidemics not all protests were directed at government action. Government inaction, too, was becoming a source of concern among the Indian middle classes. This concern would only become more intense as the status and authority of scientific medicine grew. Members of the Indian middle class and elites began to call for higher levels of government investment in the public health and sanitary state of India, and particularly Indian cities.

By the second half of the nineteenth century, orthodox western medicine was recognized by its practitioners, sponsors, and consumers as a fundamental part of the imperial enterprise and encounter. Clearly, this close association did not necessarily render scientific medicine well liked or popular with the Indian masses. To a greater or lesser extent, the mandates of this medical system were imposed willy-nilly upon an unwilling or unconvinced population. Resentment of such imperial officiousness, however, did not blind Indians to the benefits of some forms and aspects of western medicine, or to its close association with the increasingly powerful touchstones of 'modernity' and 'scientificity'.

Could this tension—between the Janus faces of colonial medicine as imposed and yet desired, exotically attractive and yet dangerously foreign—help to explain what contemporaries saw as an Indian enthusiasm for *western* medical alternatives? Two examples will allow us to explore this question: both mesmerism and homeopathy experienced periods of high visibility and apparent popularity in colonial India, just as both systems were facing increasing hostility from the orthodox profession in Europe and North America. The systems do share a number of attributes apparently favourable to their acceptance in India: both, as we saw in Chapter 2, maintained the patient's position at the centre of the therapeutic encounter, and strong commitments to idiosyncrasy and the dynamic relationship between bodies and their social and physical environments—key tropes of Ayurveda and Unani Tibb. Neither was as harsh, or as deeply committed, as scientific medicine to enforcing the exclusivity of medical professional's ability to read and interpret the body's signs. But despite these similarities, the cases of mesmerism and homeopathy in India are in important ways quite different.

The story of mesmerism in India illustrates the complex relationship between medicine and what has become known as orientalism.[15] Put simply, 'orientalism' designates an approach to scholarly, political, and social understanding that defines 'the East' as the opposite of 'the West'—as everything 'the West' is not. Thus if, as the Victorians certainly believed, western nations and cultures (or at least Britain) could be defined as rational, analytical, scientific, informed, modern, active, striving, and inherently masculine, then India (and other Asian societies) was necessarily irrational, superstitious, mystical, ignorant, traditional, passive, stagnating, and feminine—or worse, effeminate. Because Europeans expected India and Indians to exhibit these traits, they tended to see them everywhere. This in turn meant that Indian resistance to new policies or practices could always be blamed on slavish loyalty to tradition, superstition, and intransigent ignorance. Often, too, westerners assumed that appealing to these 'oriental' qualities would be an effective way to address and persuade an Indian audience.

When European mesmerism first appeared on the subcontinent in the 1840s, its principal advocate followed exactly this approach in his quest to popularize mesmerism amongst Indians (and render its use, at least on Indian bodies, acceptable to officials and the Anglo-Indian community). James Esdaile, a Scottish surgeon, was already running the Native Hospital in a village on the periphery of Calcutta when he first encountered mesmerism. After either reading an English account of mesmerism, or hearing about it from a friend (his accounts differ slightly on this point), he almost immediately tried the technique on one of the men under his care—a jailed Indian criminal. Having successfully removed the mesmerically anaesthetized man's scrotal tumour in front of a hurriedly assembled group of British observers, Esdaile was unsurprisingly impressed and enthused. He mesmerized more patients, recruited more witnesses of higher social standing, and repeated his miracle of painless surgery.

While deploying science and socially prominent witness-converts to reach out to the Anglo-Indian community on whom his position and hopes for professional advancement depended, Esdaile did not neglect the indigenous elites, or the wider population from which his patients were drawn. However, he reached out to them very differently, using the language of magic and mysticism, and presenting himself as a 'brother magician'. He insisted that his patients should be kept unaware of the mesmeric process, and be treated 'in a state of nature' if at all possible. Moreover, he and his fellow enthusiasts were eager to draw attention to India's own 'charmers' or 'medical conjurors', who, their British counterparts asserted, were practising an archaic version of mesmerism customary in India from 'time immemorial':

Doctor Strong one day asked me . . . if there was any reason to suppose that the natives of this country knew mesmerism before we introduced it among them. I replied that it could not reasonably be doubted, and that their medical conjurers are often genuine mesmerisers . . . This has been confirmed from different quarters, and especially by Dr. Davidson, late resident at Jeyepore. This gentleman, visiting our hospital and seeing the mesmerizers stroking and breathing upon the patients, said 'I now understand what the "*jar-phoonk*" of Upper India means; it is nothing but mesmerism.' Being requested to explain himself, he continued:—'Many of my people, after I had tried in vain to cure them of different severe complaints, used to ask leave for several weeks to be treated by the *Jadoo-wallah*, or conjurer; and to my great surprise, they often returned quite well, and, in reply to my enquiries, they always said that they had undergone a process called "*jar-phoonk*" I could never understand what this was, but now I see is before me; it is the combination of stroking and breathing; "*jarna*" being to *stroke*, and "*phoonka*" to *breathe*; which very correctly describes the mesmeric process.'[16]

Thus mesmerism was given an ancient pedigree, while Indian healing practices were simultaneously depicted as primitive versions of sophisticated western ones, tainted by the mystifications of their practitioners.

Esdaile was trying to accomplish three tasks with his use of mesmerism in India. Immediately, he sought to popularize mesmerism amongst Indians both to enhance the appeal of western medicine generally, and to render such Indian patients as came under his care compliant and readily treatable. He wished also to gain official sanction for mesmerism's medical use in Indian hospitals, dispensaries, and other official institutions. Finally—but perhaps most importantly to Esdaile himself—he was determined to prove the value and validity of mesmerism to the orthodox medical community in Britain, by demonstrating its efficacy, morality, and safety: 'my sole object' he later wrote,

has been to *unite* and *not to dissociate* mesmerism from medicine,…my constant aim has been to add this new healing knowledge to what we already possess, being painfully oppressed with a sense of the *miserable impotency of our present resources in combating the host of evils that human flesh is heir to.*

Esdaile succeeded, albeit to a limited extent, in his first two goals. Having gone over the heads of his medical peers in Calcutta to directly recruit the interest and support of the regional government, Esdaile succeeded in persuading officials to give him a hospital in which to demonstrate mesmeric medicine and surgery for a trial period of one year. At the end of this period, the trials had been attended by sufficient publicity (much of it carefully orchestrated by Esdaile himself) and therapeutic success to garner for mesmerism considerable public approval, and for Esdaile a new title and position: Presidency Surgeon. The experimental hospital, however, was closed, on the grounds that Indians should become self-sufficient, and fund such an institution themselves should they deem it worthy. Enough Indians of higher social standing took up the cause of mesmerism to do exactly that, and funded a voluntary mesmeric practice based in a charity dispensary, but rather grandly titled the Mesmeric Hospital in Calcutta. Esdaile's efforts to get mesmerism official approval and standing reaped a similarly limited harvest. On the positive side, he had persuaded high-ranking officials—even the Governor General of India, the Marquis of Dalhousie—that mesmeric anaesthesia at least was a genuine phenomenon and could be an effective surgical technique. (It is at least an intriguing coincidence that acupuncture's twentieth-century return to the centre stage of western medicine also began with its use as a surgical anaesthetic.) He had gained permission to use mesmerism in India's hospitals; but he had not persuaded his fellow doctors that mesmerism was practical as a hospital procedure or effective on Europeans; nor had he convinced the wider European and Indian lay elites that it was morally or socially acceptable. The Mesmeric Hospital opened in 1848; Esdaile himself retired and returned to Britain in 1851. The Hospital closed before the end of the next decade, drained of the funds and support it had attracted in the spotlight of Esdaile's well-oiled publicity machine.

In Esdaile's final and most heartfelt endeavour, the struggle to gain acceptance for mesmerism among the British profession, he did have two crucial advantages, both stemming directly from his colonial setting and patient base. First, the population he was entrancing could, in British eyes, very appropriately fall under his sway. Second, British assumptions about Indians, and the non-white races in general, lent credibility to Esdaile's assertions that his patients could not be disruptively complicit in their treatment. The historian and parliamentarian Thomas Babington Macaulay had already defined Bengalis for educated Britons as enfeebled, effeminate, and 'thoroughly fitted by nature and by habit for the foreign yoke'.[17] Esdaile's experiments merely confirmed Macaulay's vision, and demonstrated its effects in the medical sphere.

The people of this part of the world seem to be particularly sensitive to the mesmeric power; and as it has been observed that a depressed state of the nervous system favours its reception, we can easily observe why they, as a body, should be more easily affected than Europeans. Taking the population of Bengal generally, they are a feeble, ill-nourished race, remarkably deficient in nervous energy . . . Their mental constitution also favours us; we have none of the morbid irritability of the nerve, and the mental impatience of the civilised man to contend against; both of which resist and neutralise the efforts of nature.

Indians, he concluded, were 'simple, unsophisticated children of nature; neither thinking, questioning, nor remonstrating, but passively submitting to my pleasure, without in the least understanding my object or intentions . . .'.[18] And if they could not think, act, or understand, then surely, unlike their British counterparts, they could not deceive. Consider, for example, Esdaile's comment on his first mesmerically anaesthetized patient: 'it was morally and physically impossible that the man could be an impostor, inasmuch as he could not imitate what he had never heard of; . . . as the man could not possibly imagine what was expected, there could be no imagination at work . . . '.[19] So mesmerism was not as socially destabilizing or morally disruptive when practised in India, on Indians. By the same token, however, mesmerism's critics and doubters—and even its supporters—were also at liberty to regard Indian results as non-transferable. The Marquis of Dalhousie, for example, offered little support for the use of mesmerism in Britain, despite his role in promoting its use in India. When approached by the Poor Law Guardians of Exeter to advise them in their deliberations over the use of mesmerism in their lunatic asylum, Dalhousie replied:

Of the efficacy of Dr. Esdaile's practice of mesmerism in cases of lunacy I am not able to say anything. . . . Dr. Esdaile undoubtedly did possess the faculty of so influencing the sensations of natives of India by means of mesmerism, as to reduce them to a state of insensibility, not less complete than that which is now produced by the use of chloroform. . . . Whether he can influence the English constitution in the same manner or in the same degree, as he undoubtedly influenced the native constitution, I cannot pretend to say.[20]

Mesmerism was a foreign medical practice, which its importers attempted to engraft upon India through a supposedly 'oriental' rhetoric, and through uncovering Indian precursors. However, mesmerism in India was in fact practised under government auspices, by Government appointees and their Indian subordinates. It was largely practised upon lower caste charity patients with few if any other medical options, and no control over their own treatment once admitted to hospital. It was deliberately used by its chief advocate to create wards full of disciplined bodies—quiet, passive, and easily managed patients, amenable to and available for any medical procedure because entranced. So although mesmerism was certainly fiercely opposed and equally ferociously defended as an alternative system in Britain, in India it acted as a traditional tool of empire. Esdaile and his successors had no desire to integrate their technique with India's own medical traditions: far from it. Even while acknowledging the resemblance between mesmerism and certain traditional practices (and calling upon that resemblance to argue for a model of mesmerism as a natural force), colonial mesmerists actively denied those traditional forms of practice any recognition as 'medicine'. Instead, they were denigrated as 'magic' or 'superstition' or 'mysticism'. Indians were trained to mesmerize, but only as subalterns; their practice of mesmerism, like that of their compatriots outside the hospital, was rigorously defined as non-medical, in this case because merely mechanical.

Practised most visibly in imperial institutions, disconnected from its Indian context, with little to offer Indians in terms of status, recognition, or increased agency as patients, and few points of cross-cultural contact—for voluntary hospitals could serve only a minority of patients, and the technique was deemed too time-intensive for the public hospitals—mesmerism could never offer Indians an alternative to orthodox western medicine. Meanwhile, the very responsiveness of Indians to mesmerism was used as evidence of their 'oriental' proclivities, their 'racial' debility, and their inferior physical and mental endowments. As such, even the most positive evidence from India—for example, Esdaile's successful removal under mesmeric anaesthesia of a tumour 7 feet in circumference and weighing 103 pounds from a patient who himself only weighed 114 pounds—could only confirm mesmerism's heterodoxy in Britain, reconfiguring it as an exotic treatment suitable only for exotic diseases and exotically inferior bodies.

Homeopathy, arriving in India slightly earlier, but initially in the same place (Bengal), presents a very different picture of western heterodoxy in a non-western and cross-cultural context. Its passage to India was sped by soldiers, missionaries, traders, medical speculators and homeopathic converts from across the European continent—in other words, by an eclectic and widely dispersed array of supporters. Individuals did not have to be medically trained to read Hahnemann's *Organon*, or to purchase an appropriate selection of homeopathic remedies. In fact, creative homeopathic entrepreneurs across Europe were soon selling kits specifically designed for outward-bound colonists and empire-builders. The rising popularity of homeopathy was noted by the Anglo-Indian press, one journal observing in 1852 that homeopathy was 'extensively practiced by amateurs, in the civil and military services'. By the very nature of empire, enthusiasts in these two groups were to be found in even the most remote outposts of empire. The same author noted that as a result, '[there is] scarcely a large district in India in which such an amateur has not for years been diffusing benefits around him.'[21] These logistical advantages, independent of the medical and doctrinal content of the homeopathic system, made it far easier for homeopathy than for either allopathy or mesmerism to recruit support among Indians themselves. Moreover, purely as a consumer good, homeopathy was ideally tailored to meet the needs and tastes of the emerging and influential *bhadralok* (or 'respectable people'): homeopathy's principal text, the *Organon*, was readily available in English and vernacular translations and had been written initially for lay audiences; the medicines prescribed were similarly obtainable; and its treatments—mild and free from forbidden animal products and alcohol—could all be administered in the home by family members.

Moreover, as adherents to a self-proclaimed alternative system and as medical heretics, homeopathists had rapidly acquired experience in institution-building—experience which helps to explain the existence in India of at least three homeopathic hospitals by 1852. These private charitable institutions, and the many added to their number by the end of the century, were 'modern' and 'western'—but they were not imperial. The rancorous debates between homeopaths and allopaths had left little room for confusion about the exclusion of homeopathy from the institutions of western orthodoxy, whether at home or in the colonies. Those debates—and in passing, considerable knowledge about the practice of homeopathy—were transmitted to India largely through the medium of the medical press. The quarterly *Journal of the Calcutta Medical and Physical Society*, for example, devoted its summer issue to reprinting a range of articles on homeopathy recently published in the British medical press. They started with the transcript of William Kingdon's speech to the Medical Society of London. This selection is suggestive: as we saw in Chapter 2, Kingdon was a regularly trained practitioner, and initially highly sceptical of homeopathic doctrine. His oration, beginning as it did with a description of his own introduction to the practice through the demands of his patients, would have had resonated strongly with readers in India. First, his demanding—but respected and respectable—patients would immediately have reminded medical readers of their own paying patients, and lay readers of themselves. His initial disbelief in the face of homeopathy's 'naked absurdity' was balanced by his call to experiment:

[I]f any good arise out of this system, it must be such as is competent to overcome all the preconceived notions of the proper use of medicine . . . I could hardly respect that mind which would grant credence to such a proposition without experimenting for itself. No more can I respect those feelings which would characterise as knaves or fools a large body of industrious individuals, rather than take the trouble to investigate into the truth of their assertions.[22]

Kingdon's acceptance of homeopathic efficacy was gradual, entirely pragmatic, and strictly empirical. Most importantly in relation to the Indian context, it was partial and contingent.

I am not at present a homeopath, nor do I feel as if I ever should be. I cannot forgo the auxilliaries of the lancet, leeches, or the cupping-glass . . . which in many cases I know to be certainly beneficial, and impossible to be injurious, for any new plan; but where there is great uncertainty, or where, though medicine may be applicable to the disease it may be of a nature to injure the constitution, there I should feel authorised, with close watchfulness to treat cases upon a system that cannot possibly do harm.[23]

All in all, Kingdon's contribution was a call to adaptation and to pragmatic adoption of any cure, from any system, if it worked. It was a call well suited to the particular conditions of medicine in India: its pluralism, its uncontrolled and apparently uncontrollable epidemics, and the desperate conditions of its urban and especially rural poor.

The *Journal* followed it with four more articles reprinted from the British medical press, filled with biting sarcasm and repudiations of homeopathy as outright fraud and quackery. But these articles were tailored to an exclusively British and exclusively medical audience. The poisonously adversarial nature of the debate looked very different to observers accustomed to a pluralistic medical culture. One western-trained Indian doctor commented that in India,

there is no need for anyone to set up a sect of his own, and proclaim from the housetops: 'There is only one way to sound health, and that is my way; follow me if you are wise and so save yourself.' But with our Western brethren, the case seems to be quite different. There we have an ever-increasing number of medical sects, each with a special nostrum or formula wherewith to cure or charm away all ills that flesh is heir to. Each may undoubtedly have its own limited field of usefulness . . . but the danger is in the attempt to transform it into a universal panacea. The rate at which specialists of this type are increasing is truly appalling. One would cure all ills by osteopathy, another by chromopathy, another by homeopathy, a fourth by allopathy, others by electricity, baths, food reform, vaccine-therapy, charms, incantation, miracle workings, magnetic healing . . . the list goes on till one fails to see the forest for the trees . . . It is only natural that under such circumstances, a sort of distrust of all specialists is created in the popular mind.[24]

Advertently or not, the overall tone of orthodox medicine's combative contributions to the Indian debate encouraged experiment with homeopathy, if only because of the general distrust engendered by their insistence on exclusivity.

And many in India did experiment—including regularly trained Indian physicians, like Mahendralal Sircar, whose initial denunciations of homeopathy rendered all the more spectacular his conversion. Mahendralal's defection was revealing in another way: he was, and continued after his homeopathic turn to be, a vocal proponent of science and 'scientific' medicine, founding in 1867 the Indian Association for the Cultivation of Science to promote the growth of an indigenous scientific community, and the creation of scientific knowledge by and for Indians.[25] He promoted homeopathy through the *Calcutta Journal of Medicine* he founded a year later, as a scientific and modern system. The *Journal*'s slogan was a verse from the *Caraka Samhita*: 'That alone is the right medicine which can remove disease; He alone is the true physician who can restore health', and this pragmatic, empirical, but certainly rational approach characterized both the publication and broadly, the Indian approach to homeopathy.[26] Alongside the ease with which homeopathy could be accessed by laymen and aspiring professionals, its self-proclaimed allegiance to science was a major attraction, particularly to the educated middle classes. Moreover, its visible programme of experimentation—drug 'provings'—was one of relatively few routes towards participation in the scientific endeavour accessible to Indians. Until the 1890s and 1900s, when the Indian Medical Service became more open to Indian 'regulars', it was not uncommon for men like Mahendralal—trained in orthodox medicine, and committed to science—to turn to homeopathy. They faced substantial obstacles of race, class, and economics to an allopathic career: the Indian Medical Service was reluctant to employ and promote Indian doctors; the private practice of western medicine was fiercely competitive, with an increasing number of 'regulars' chasing the business of the Anglo-Indian community; and the cost-barriers to allopathy were high, both for would-be doctors (who had to pay for their educations) and willing patients. Homeopathy offered an easier entrée to 'modern' medical knowledge and practice with its higher status and often higher fees.

On grounds of access, affordability, and potential for advancement, then, homeopathy was attractive to individual consumers and practitioners alike; in terms of politics, homeopathy was chosen, rather than imposed, and brought Indians into an international community as equals. But what of creed? Was there anything in the homeopathic system itself—from *similia similibus curantur* to the doctrine of infinitesimals—that rendered it particularly suitable to India in a way that mesmerism and allopathy were not? Observers then and scholars now have argued that homeopathy was easier to 'indigenize' or vernacularize (though obviously the willingness of European homeopaths to accept Indians as colleagues would certainly have fostered this impression, independently of the intellectual content of the system). In 1882, the editor of the *Indian*

Medical Gazette asserted that 'the mystery of homeopathy rather commends itself to the native mind'; others noted that Hahnemann himself had studied 'the fragmentary medical lore of the older India' as he constructed his system, and that therefore Ayurveda and homeopathy were kindred systems.[27] More tangibly, homeopathy's supporters were far more willing to engage with Ayurveda and Ayurvedic practitioners, regarding their expertise as a national resource. Homeopathists, like hakims and *vaidyas*, were also highly critical of the brutality, the inhumanity, the materialist and generalizing tendencies, and the professional and doctrinal arrogance of allopathy. However, the modernizers who turned to homeopathy as a rational alternative to orthodox western medicine cherished no illusions about the merits of Ayurveda and Unani Tibb; both of the traditional systems would have to change, and take into account the discoveries of modern medicine. Nonetheless, homeopathy demonstrated a different model of what a 'modern' medical system could look like: it was more humane, and even more scientific (because based on a set of predictive laws, like physics).

Medically, homeopathy also had something to offer that was uniquely suited to India: as well as palatable and affordable treatments for the many minor complaints ignored by public health officers and government dispensaries, homeopathy claimed to have discovered treatments for two major diseases that continued to baffle its allopathic competition—cholera and malaria. Whether or not the homeopathic remedies cured cholera, they were certainly no less effective than their allopathic counterparts, and were considerably kinder. And of course it was his experiments with the effects of quinine (then the most effective treatment for malaria) that Hahnemann credited with inspiring homeopathy in the first place.

Homeopathy, then, thrived in India in part because it was not intrinsically opposed to Indian culture and medical traditions. Untainted by a too-close association with an often high-handed and insensitive bureaucracy, homeopathy was 'scientific' without being sanctioned. Both in relation to science and in relation to nationalism, homeopathy allowed middle-class Indians in particular to reverse the polarity of colonial medical stereotypes. They could be doctors rather than patients; active experimentalists rather than passive subjects; modernizers rather than traditionalists. Moreover, homeopathy was rational, culturally free-floating—it was practised in India by Europeans and Indians alike, and was not identified with any particular nation—and required no change of world view.

Thus far I've examined Indian responses to systems peripheral or running counter to the medical mainstream in the West; nor was either mesmerism or homeopathy central to the imperial endeavour. But of course, medicine itself was at the heart of empire, or at least pinned firmly to Britannia's ample bosom, a merit badge for her 'civilizing' efforts. And 'medicine' as a system of thought, a body of knowledge, a set of tools, and a professional discipline was in flux. The laboratory and germ theory, emerging at this time as new foci and forces for medical change, threatened to undo the unifying effects of homeopathy and other alternative threats. They also challenged the basis for some of medicine's claims to authority in social and moral matters. For example, where humouralist, miasmic views of health enabled the Sanitarians to imbue moral truths and social assumptions with medical force, germs as disease causes were apparently blind to race, creed, and class. Within the profession, the claims made by promoters of the laboratory, that lab tests were the most reliable basis for diagnosis of an increasing number of diseases, were seen as threatening to the status of the bedside clinician, and the intimacy of the doctor–patient relationship. If a doctor could not definitively name at the bedside, by observing and questioning the patient, the disease from which its occupant suffered, without relying on a faceless technician totally unaware of the patient's particular circumstances, then how would patients be able to trust in medical authority? Both germ theory and the labs that put it into practice played active and highly visible roles in imperialism, and in India. So how did Indians respond to this form of cross-cultural medicine, embedded in and imbued with all the assumptions of imperialism—but also contested, scrutinized, and from the perspective of the nineteenth-century world, profoundly counter-intuitive?

Temperate Seeds in Tropical Soils: Germ Theory in the Indian Medical Marketplace

William Osler remarked in 1905 that

The quarrels of doctors make a pretty chapter in the history of medicine. Each generation seems to have had its own. The Coans and Cnidians, the Arabians and the Galenists, the Brunonians and the Broussonians, the Homeopaths and the Regulars, have in different centuries, rent the robe of Aesculapius

and of course the bald statement that 'doctors differ' is a truism applied to non-western and western practitioners alike.[28] But as we've seen, since at least the seventeenth century practitioners in South Asia were perceived by westerners as 'differing' far less, in their basic understandings of diseases and in their practices, from their European counterparts.

Perhaps the competitive and pluralistic medical marketplaces of South Asia acted to unify—at least in scholarly rhetoric—proponents of each of its major medical systems in the same way that the battle against homeopathy united European and North American 'regulars' of all stripes. Or perhaps—and more likely—this perceived homogeneity simply exemplifies the Orientalist vision of a monolithic and unchanging 'timeless East'. In any case, when the rise of germ theory and 'scientific medicine' (like homeopathy and mesmerism before them) threatened the fragile unity of the western profession, Indian traditional practitioners took careful note of the debates that followed.

One of the more famous anecdotes of the germ-theory era exemplifies both the timing and public nature of the debate involved. The story is that of Max Von Pettenkofer, an eminent Bavarian hygienist and public health worker. In the 1890s, debate raged within the medical and public health communities across Europe about whether any disease could be caused by an external agent (often analogized to a 'seed') alone, or whether such agents, although necessary, were not in themselves sufficient to produce a disease, but only acted on an already debilitated body (analogized to the 'soil'). Robert Koch, pre-eminent scientist of the germ, had recently isolated an organism that he asserted was the sole and exclusive cause of

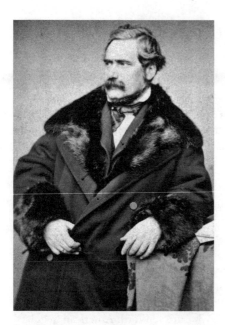

19. Max Josef von Pettenkofer, c.1860s.

cholera. Proponents of the germ school were anxious to make this discovery grounds for the triumph of their disease model. Pettenkofer, meanwhile, continued to declare his deep scepticism of the gospel of germs and argued that no one in good health could be sickened by a germ alone, in the absence of an unsanitary environment, poor nutrition, hereditary defect, or other factors. Dramatically, he illustrated his contempt for 'germs' by downing a glass of water liberally inoculated with the specimen of cholera vibrio recently sent to him from Koch's own laboratory. Notably, Pettenkofer experienced diarrhoea (which he investigated microscopically and found to be full of the putative cholera bacilli) but no substantial ill effects from his unusual tipple. He thus illustrated to his own satisfaction the importance of the 'soil' (the patient's own constitution) in the advent of disease.[29]

Although notions of contagion were widely accepted in this period, the idea of germs as the sole effective agents of that contagion took considerable time to become orthodoxy. Only in the 1890s and 1900s were medical students in Europe and North

America consistently encouraged to see 'germs' wherever they saw communicable disease. And even then, their convictions and arguments were still couched in terms of faith as much as in terms of science. Germs remained dogmatic as well as experimental entities; indeed, one doctor echoed the catechism in expressing his own allegiance to germ theory:

I hold that every contagious disease is caused by the introduction into the system of a living organism or microzyme, capable of reproducing its kind, and minute beyond all reach of sense. I hold that as all life on our planet is the result of antecedent life, so is all specific disease the result of antecedent specific disease. I hold that as no germ can originate *de novo*, neither can a scarlet fever come into existence spontaneously. I hold that as an oak comes from an oak, a grape from a grape, so does a typhoid fever come from a typhoid germ, a diphtheria from a diphtheria germ; and that a scarlatina could no more proceed from a typhoid germ that could a sea-gull from a pigeon's egg.[30]

Germ theory had to compete with older explanations of epidemic and endemic disease, explanations that had already proven their power to prevent illness. Predominant among these were miasmatic and zymotic models. Both of these systems of explanation blamed disease on filth, pollution, and contamination, with their sequelae of stench, poor air quality, and decay/putrefaction; miasma, the older of the two was, in the simplest terms, a view that bad air, arising from decay and fermentation in an unclean environment, caused disease; zymotic theory glossed 'miasma' in terms of particulate decayed matter, spreading in the air and water, and contaminating all they touched, thus catalysing the internal disease process. Conversely, fresh air and sunlight, in conjunction with clean, moral, and well-nourished bodies, were the acme of disease prevention in both models. Neither enrolled the notion of 'specific disease'—rather, each retained notions of idiosyncrasy, in which the particular illnesses developed by contaminated individuals depended upon their own constitutions and habits, and the environments around them. Combined with poverty, ignorance, and immorality, the 'filth' factors were the targets of lay and medical public health campaigners, who operated under the banner of Sanitarianism. The Sanitarians sought to prevent particularly urban disease by cleansing cities of their disease-ridden grime, improving the housing stock, providing clean water, educating and morally reforming the poor, and harnessing the new sciences of statistics and hygiene to quantify and improve the public health. Using statistics, Sanitarians could prove that their methods, expensive, and time-consuming though they were, worked—and worked to produce not merely purer environments and healthier cities, but what they saw as a more moral and more Christian culture as well. These were the models that germ theory had either to displace or to co-opt, if it was to become the primary mode of understanding health and disease.

Britain's colonies were regarded by her 'germ-enthusiasts' and proponents of 'scientific medicine' as essential laboratories for the proving and deployment of germ theory. With scientific progress increasingly seen as an emblem of national prominence, even a wealth of germs could become grounds for nationalistic pride and competitiveness. As a *Lancet* editorial of 1895, reporting on the Indian Medical Congress of the preceding year, observed,

Crombie [President of the Medical Section of the Indian Medical Congress] concluded his excellent address with an appeal to his medical hearers in Calcutta not to allow France and Germany to remain in the van of bacteriological research, but to make more careful study of the cases which came under their observation in India...what is wanted is...work by trained experts in properly equipped laboratories to supplement the clinical work of medical officers....In this way scientific and practical work would go hand in hand and some real progress would be made. India presents a rich field for investigations of this nature.[31]

Yet even the *Lancet*'s aggressively germ-theorist—and hardly mealy-mouthed—editors were obliged to add a caveat:

The fact that Koch's comma bacillus for example is present in cases of cholera may be taken as established; but its causal connexion with cholera has, in the opinion of many, still to be demonstrated as an adequate explanation of all the phenomena of that disease as it comports itself in Indian experience. These and many other questions in Eastern medicine and pathology are still awaiting solution, and India affords a wide field for their investigation by the aid of modern methods and appliances of pathological and bacteriological research[32]

The way this passage uses the phrase 'Eastern medicine and pathology' is suggestive of the changing stature of orthodox medicine (at least in the eyes of its defenders and practitioners): 'Eastern medicine' no longer refers to the medical systems indigenous to India; instead, it refers to orthodox western medicine—biomedicine—as practised in 'Eastern' climes. Was this merely a casual use of language, or did it indicate a conviction that medicine as practised in the West was universal? Such usage was common, and the conflation of western medicine with 'medicine' writ large—relegating all other systems to the status of mere 'witch-doctoring', 'conjuring', or 'custom'—was a commonplace. Of course, the passage also reiterates its metropolitan author's view of India as fertile soil for the cultivation of scientific medicine.

Some members of the colonial medical elites on the ground were eager to demonstrate the efficacy and efficiency of health policies informed by germ theory—and thus to assert the new power and authority of medicine. Others saw such policies as simply perpetuating under a different name the Sanitarian model of public health, with its linkage between disease and morality: a particularly fraught connection in the colonies' non-Christian societies. And many feared germ theory and models of public health based upon it as potential sources of social, economic, and political disruption. Germ theory, as we saw in the case of plague, located the invisible, intangible, and yet highly contagious source of disease within the bodies of individuals—and meant that programmes of disease prevention were necessarily going to become very intimate indeed. Imperial authorities knew that enforcing such intimacy surveillance posed endless risks of cultural offence. At the same time, focusing on individual bodies threatened some programmes that were popular with powerful interests in India—expensive programmes of urban sanitation, for example, initially intended to create healthier cities by removing miasma. Like Pettenkofer's dramatic swigging of germs, the debates

between these groups were explicitly intended for public consumption—
and they extended well into the twentieth century.

Amongst that public in India were, of course, many well-educated
and active healers and consumers of the indigenous medical systems,
whether Unani Tibb, Siddha, or Ayurveda. Such colonial subjects
were not only well aware of contemporary medical debates, but
actively used the arguments put forward by European critics of
scientific medicine to support education and training in traditional
medical systems. Essentially, proponents of India's own medical
systems selectively assimilated those aspects of germ theory that
were consistent with their own systems—while using the conten-
tion and discord within western medicine to justify discarding less
readily digestible elements. Traces of this very selective adoption of
western scientific knowledge are clearly visible in official documents, like the remarkable *Report of the Committee on the Indigenous
Systems of Medicine, Madras*—also known as the *Usman* (or sometimes *Uthman*) *Report* after the Committee's Chairman Khan Baha-
dur Muhammad Usman, a prominent member of the Madras
Legislative Council.

The *Report* is important in part because of its timing. It was
commissioned in 1921, reflecting the greater powers granted to
elected Indian members of provincial parliaments. After two years
of gruelling work by committee members, it was published in 1923.
In other words, it appeared as germ theory was achieving the status
of established orthodoxy in the West, but also just after one of its
most severe and public tests—the influenza pandemic of 1918–19.
In Europe, some parts of the medical community remained am-
bivalent: they plumped for germs, but hedged their bets. The
British, for example, continued to build pavilion hospitals and
Nightingale wards (both of which were designed to fight disease
as it was conceptualized by sanitarian and miasmatic, *not* germ
theory, models—via eliminating filth and putrefaction, not mi-
crobes) until the 1930s. On the front lines of the new science
of bacteriology, meanwhile, its adherents were building a more
sophisticated and integrated model in which both 'seed' and 'soil'
were essential to disease aetiology. The germ remained the 'seed',

but the 'soil' was generally construed as the individual human body, rather than the wider environment.[33]

Moreover, the *Usman Report* was written in the wake of aggressive attempts by practitioners of western medicine in India to undermine the practice and privileges of other systems. Between 1912 and 1917, Indian healers of all denominations witnessed the passage of the Medical Acts establishing India's Medical Councils and medical registers. Both the Councils and the registers excluded practitioners of any of the indigenous systems. Yet it was from these registers that medical appointment holders had to be drawn—in effect, mandating a monopoly for western medicine in any government-funded institution or position. The Acts were subsequently used to justify removing from the Register even western practitioners convicted of association with Ayurvedic or Unani practitioners, in much the same way that British and American medical associations had punished regulars for consulting with homeopathic colleagues.

In the course of their study, the committee elicited responses to a detailed questionnaire from 183 'native practitioners' writing in eight different languages; personally interviewed forty of these respondents; and delegated a subcommittee to tour India, examining at first hand medical practices, schools, and centres of indigenous medical learning. Moreover, the Committee pursued a broad remit, having been commissioned to 'afford the exponents of the Ayurvedic and Unani systems the opportunity to state their case fully in writing for scientific criticism and to justify State encouragement of these systems'.[34] In other words, this committee was to address questions both of the systems' medical worth and efficacy, and of whether they were worthy of state support, recognition, and encouragement. And it was to be composed of 'non-official gentlemen' representing all of the systems under scrutiny, as well as western medicine. Moreover, Madras granted the committee its requested—and fairly substantial—budget of 30,000 rupees (not including the salaries of its secretary and chair) for the first six months alone—an amount which was apparently renewed several times over the life of the Committee. That the report, and the method by which it was compiled, was influential is visible in the fact that it became the Indian Medical Service's chosen model

for future inquiries into the value of State support for and responsibility to indigenous medicine. This influence seems to have persisted
as late as the *1948–1949 Report of the Committee on Indigenous Systems of
Medicine* (Chopra Committee), a report that takes a similar shape—
though without quite the same mission of offering a 'scientific
critique' and assessment of the systems under study.[35]

The Committee responsible for the *Usman Report* shared with their
many predecessors the perception of Indian medicine as more unified
than its western counterpart, and regarded that unity as a positive
attribute. They fostered this view in their discussions, drawing attention to 'the common foundations of all these three schools' and
proposing 'to consider them as one triune whole'.[36] Even more
explicitly, the committee's secretary tartly noted: 'Certainly there
has been less exhibition in Ayurveda than in Western medicine of
too hasty a promulgation of new and novel theories followed by their
subsequent repudiation, and of that alternate enunciation and denun-
ciation of hypotheses which is sometimes mistaken for progress.'[37]
At least in some eyes, then, a slower rate of medical change could be a
healthy sign, rather than evidence of a hidebound dependence on
tradition. Committee members also made a point of noting the deep
divisions in western medicine, and in particular commented extensively on those between homeopaths and allopaths, and between
those who supported laboratory methods and those who privileged,
instead, clinical experience and observation in diagnosis.
  Several members of the committee also critiqued the imperial
tendency towards the purely extractive study of indigenous medicine:

There are many well-meaning persons . . . [who] are nevertheless of the
opinion that it is not necessary to study the science of Indian medicine to
know the use of these remedial measures, and that practitioners of western
medicine may be well-trusted to use them in the light of their own
pathology, diagnosis, and the like; they are ready to incorporate into
their pharmacopoeia such of these indigenous drugs and methods of
treatment which are found efficient in practice, but have no patience
with the rest of the Indian systems themselves; in other words, they
would take in the art, but would shut out the science . . . [38]

Strikingly, this passage equates indigenous medical cosmologies and theory with science (and certainly they played equivalent roles in ordering medical perceptions of the world and were equally rooted in the organized study and interpretation of the phenomena of the natural world). The analogy with which the authors continue is equally apt and equally pointed:

Such use of indigenous drugs and remedial measures would be as unscientific and dangerous a quackery as, for instance, the use of vaccines, sera, and hypodermic remedies by Ayurvedists who have not learned the science on which their use is based, though, by a little practice, they may easily learn the art of hypodermic or even intravenous injections.[39]

In the extensive appendices to the *Report*, Srinivasamurti and the chairman of its Urdu subcommittee offered more detailed analyses of 'the science and art of Indian medicine', beginning with the vexed question of whether or not the Indian systems were 'scientific'.[40] Srinivasamurti, himself western-trained and a self-declared 'devotee' of western science, spent considerable time explaining Indian science to his western audience. He unpicked faulty assumptions—for instance, that the *dosas* were straightforwardly equivalent to the Greek humours, (see the Introduction, above, for similarities and differences). He also illustrated the ways in which Indian notions of matter and mind, and of the unity of science, religion, and philosophy *were* equivalent to the latest discoveries of the western hard sciences. In this mode, Srinivasamurti lingered over Freud and 'dream-states', and the likeness between the Panchabuta theory of matter (which he translates not as 'earth', 'water', 'light', 'air', and 'sky', but as 'solid', 'liquid', 'radiant', 'gaseous', and 'ethereal' states) and particle physics. Similarly, he uses the new discovery of blood groups and types to argue for the idea of *prakriti*—that in terms of body type, metabolism, and temperament, all people fall into one of three groups, *vattala*, *pithala*, and *shleshmala*.[41]

However, when Srinivasamurti turns to the question of disease causation, the impact of western medical controversies becomes explicit. He focuses closely on germ theory, and in particular on its advocates' still controversial claims about its novelty and explanatory self-sufficiency. Arguing that Ayurveda already possessed a concept of germ-causation, he claimed simply that such a model 'did not, and does not occupy in Ayurveda that all-important position which it does in modern western medicine.'[42] Rather, in Ayurveda,

[The] germ-seed is merely one among the many external causative factors of disease, . . . and there does not seem to be any special reason why the germ alone should be assigned a unique and all-important role . . . This fact is, in a way, recognized by western medicine also; . . . although some germ enthusiasts are hard at work to find out causative germs for all diseases in general; it is because of the undue importance attached to germs, that it sometimes appears as though germ-theory was the whole of our Western theory of causation of diseases, while the fact is that it is but one among the many theories known to western medicine . . . [43]

Srinivasamurti then addressed the specific cases of cholera and tuberculosis, diseases closely identified with germ theory, the new public health—and with medically justified compulsion in both Europe and European colonies (compulsion which met with strong public resistance and condemnation in both places):

[E]ven in the case of diseases like cholera and tuberculosis, which are definitely stated to be due to specific bacteria, the chain of evidence is by no means so strong as it is generally stated to be. The germ-enthusiasts say that the cholera or tubercule bacterium is the causative agent, while the Ayurvedist will perhaps say that it is due to a particular variety of deranged doshas. Can the germ enthusiast say definitively that the cholera vibrio or tubercule bacillus is *everything* in the causation of cholera or tuberculosis? If one hundred people are exposed to the same infection, it does not follow that all will contract the disease; in addition, to the bacteria, you require a particular condition of the tissues . . . ; some hold that there are yet other factors which should be present before a person can contract the disease; let us for a moment confine ourselves only to two factors, the bacterium (which the germ enthusiast calls the exciting cause) and the particular condition of the tissues (which he calls the predisposing cause). Now are we quite sure of the exact significance of these terms . . . ? Certain germs may be living for years in our intestines on terms of neutrality . . . ; but the moment something untoward happens to the intestines, they may at once grow unfriendly and declare war. Now all these years, the so-called exciting cause was there but was powerless to excite. But the moment the intestines become injured in some way our whilom friends become our foes. Why should we not call the injury to the intestines the exciting cause and the bacterium the predisposing cause? They are apparently like the seed and the soil, the father and the mother, which are both essential . . .

Srinivasamurti thus adeptly and exactly deployed arguments identical to those raised by Sanitarians and others resisting the bacteriological gospel in Europe. His next step was to assimilate/translate them into existing Ayurvedic practices and theories:

It seems as though the Tridosha theory looks at the question more from the standpoint of the soil, while the germ theory looks at it from the standpoint of the seed. 'Keep out the seed—away with all germs and you are safe'—that is the slogan of the germ-enthusiast. 'It seems impractical to keep out the germ-seeds which are ubiquitous. Therefore keep the soil in such a condition that no seeds can grow, even if it gets in there.' So urges Ayurveda.

It is no coincidence that Srinivasamurti chose these conditions as his examples of germ theory's limitations. Both TB and cholera were diseases whose proposed bacterial causation had attracted heavy—and striking—criticism. Both too were the subjects of heated public health campaigns, which focused their attentions on the disenfranchised poor. In India, as David Arnold has illustrated, medical recommendations to control cholera amongst pilgrims and tuberculosis amongst enclosed women (and their families) had been first ignored and, when implemented even in muted form, hotly contested, as interfering with religious freedom and traditional social mores.

Srinivasamurti cited numerous western critiques of germ theory— though it is notable that his collection of doubters (including the Harveian Orator James Goodheart, and Sir James MacKenzie, a prominent cardiologist and general physician) offered their remarks largely in the period between 1900 and 1914. He also cited sources from the contemporary western press, including Bernard Shaw, Morley Roberts, and an article from the London *Times* criticizing the bacteriologically focused public health campaigns of the preceding decade, and citing workplace pollution and poor nutrition as the true 'soil' of disease. His most potent ammunition, however, was drawn from germ theory's recent and bitter defeat in the face of the influenza pandemic. He raised the spectre of influenza, and the putative 'influenza bacillus', which had been blamed but was often not found in clinical cases, yet found prolifically in the sinuses of the healthy.

Thus influenza bacillus may exist and not produce disease; on the other hand, it may be absent and we may still suffer from 'influenza'. This leads to the question, 'what is the significance of a term like influenza'? Does the name denote merely a group of clinical signs and symptoms? Or does it signify that the cause is a specific germ? It is, of course, arguable that if it is not this specific germ, it must be some others; it may be so; but does this not show there is a tendency in some quarters to make a fetish of the germ theory? Does this not suggest that there is something slippery, something unsatisfactory about it all? Medicine may be right in its high heaven, but all is not well with germ theory.

In its two volumes, the *Usman Report* also includes the report of the Unani Tibb sub-committee, and many of the 183 surveys themselves. Across these responses a similar pattern emerges, in which practitioners and proponents of the various indigenous systems use both contemporary western science *and* the intense debates that scientific claims provoked in western medicine to make a case for the superiority of India's own systems. Indian responses to the germ-theory controversies shed light on the utility of science as a tool both of resistance and of advocacy for an alternative system of natural knowledge. But it also reveals the durability of doubts inspired by competing claims to scientific and medical and moral authority. And in the later twentieth century, as ever-wider communities in the West too gained access to medical and scientific controversies through increasing media attention, this kind of doubt would spark and inspire new waves of interest in both alternative and cross-cultural medical practices.

CONCLUSION: PRAGMATISM, PLURALISM, AND THE (IM)PATIENT-CONSUMER

In this volume, I have considered the phenomena of cross-cultural and alternative medicine over the course of some three and a quarter centuries, looking at examples from three continents. Counter-intuitively, perhaps, I have argued that cross-cultural medicine, which is often popularly regarded as a relatively new phenomenon emerging from the 1960s and 1970s, is in fact very old, extending back beyond the scope of this volume to the transfer of knowledge from the Egyptians to the Greeks and the Greeks to the Arabs, the Arabs to the Indians and Europeans, and so on, ad infinitum. On the other hand, this volume illustrates that 'alternative medicine' is—if neither novel nor unique to the twentieth and twenty-first centuries—still by comparison a recent development.[1] To have medical systems, theories, and practices that can properly be regarded as 'alternative', one must have a recognized, definable, and at least relatively stable orthodoxy to which they oppose themselves. Such an orthodoxy only emerged in the western medical marketplace in the nineteenth century.

So where does this leave our perception that *something* different— bigger, more global, less culturally or professionally constrained—is happening in the medical marketplace of today? Have our medical tastes, beliefs, and encounters really changed since the mid-twentieth century? What, if anything, is genuinely new?

Tiger Balm, the now ubiquitous analgesic ointment in the brightly coloured little hexagonal jar, offers us one window on what is distinctive, and what continuous in cross-cultural medicine today. Beloved of athletes, migraine sufferers, and the easily bruised, Tiger

Balm is today marketed in 100 countries, from Hammerfest, Norway to Bluff, New Zealand. Although it is a quintessentially 'Oriental' product, the largest single market in which it is sold is actually the United States where 40,000 physical outlets and an undeterminable number of websites stock the product. They range from the predictable (martial arts suppliers, Chinese markets and pharmacies) to the unexpected (supermarket chains and veterinary supply shops). Certainly, every major US pharmacy chain carries at least the balm itself, as do Boots and similar European chains; many also carry spin-off products. Global sales of Tiger Balm and associated products in 2002 topped $35 million.

The products themselves continue to be manufactured entirely in East and South-East Asia (specifically, in China, Indonesia, the Philippines, Malaysia, Singapore, Taiwan, and Thailand). In marketing terms, however, Haw Par Healthcare Limited fairly successfully makes the best of both worlds, East and West. Its corporate literature asserts: 'Tiger Balm is not an ancient Chinese concoction, but a modern efficacious medication.' But advertisements targeting English-speaking consumers describe the product rather differently:

The origins of that formula can be traced back to the time of the Chinese emperors who sought relief for aches and pains from the stresses of court hearings, and the strains of the imperial harem. The balm would have died with the dynasties had it not been for Aw Chu Kin, who breathed new life into the ancient recipe.[2]

Certainly, this is orientalism as surely as Esdaile's descriptions of himself as a 'brother magician' when addressing an Indian audience—but it is more deftly aimed at persuading western consumers to partake of Tiger Balm's exotic and imperial charms.

20. (FACING PAGE) 'Hindoo Tobacco Habit Cure', broadside, Milford, Indiana, c.1890. While the turbaned Indian and the frequent references to opium suggest the exotic, and the 'roots and herbs' hark back to traditional folk remedies around the world, the rest of this advertisement leans on the standard claims of patent medicines in the nineteenth-century west. The small print adds a perhaps inadvertent layer of irony by asserting 'Milford Drug Co., Sole manufacturers and originators of the Hindoo Tobacco Habit Cure': the remedy was as Indian as Indiana.

The Hindoo Tobacco Habit Cure is composed entirely of Roots and Herbs.

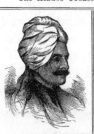

THIS IS FOR YOU!

READ IT CAREFULLY.

IF YOU DO NOT NEED THE HELP WE OFFER,

Please hand it to your neighbor. He will thank you for it.

200 DOSES 50¢

MAKES WEAK MEN STRONG.

Restores the Debilitated to Manly Vigor.

MAKES STRONG MEN STRONGER.

✳ HINDOO TOBACCO HABIT CURE ✳

The Oldest and Most Reliable Remedy on the market
for Destroying the Appetite for Tobacco
IN ALL ITS FORMS.

CHEWING, SMOKING AND CIGARETTE HABIT CURED IN TWO DAYS.

PHYSICIANS TELL YOU THERE IS NO CURE FOR THE CIGARETTE SMOKER That the entire system is so impregnated with the opium and poisons inhaled from the cigarette, and has such a firm hold on the victim that his case is hopeless. We have a positive cure in our

HINDOO REMEDY.

A FEW DOSES
DESTROYS THE APPETITE.

In two days we drive the Poison
entirely out of the system.

PERFECTLY } COMPOSED { ROOTS AND
HARMLESS, } ...ENTIRELY... OF.... { HERBS ▲ ▲ ▲

MILFORD DRUG CO.,

SOLE MANUFACTURERS AND ORIGINATORS OF THE
HINDOO TOBACCO HABIT CURE,

Milford, Indiana, U. S. A,

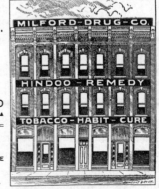

It is pleasant to take. It has cured others. It will cure you. Try it.

$500.00 to anyone who can show that we use opium, morphine, or any other harmful drugs in this remedy.

No failures when directions are followed. We have thousands of testimonials of marvelous cures. Let us have yours.

Of course, it's not our taste for the outlandish that is new. 'Ching's Chinese pills' (popular in Regency Britain), the 'Hindoo Tobacco Habit Cure' (advertised in, of all places, Indiana in the 1890s), the anti-gonorrhoic 'Gonosan' with its 'purest East Indian Sandalwood Oil and Kava-Kava resins' and hundreds of other products like them demonstrate that western consumers have eagerly sought 'oriental' cures and 'eastern' medical wisdom for centuries (see Figure 20). But those products were the medical equivalent of Chinese and Japanese export war, the plates and tea pots and lacquered screens whose 'Chinese scenes' might have been painted in Canton or printed up in Staffordshire, but in either case bore little resemblance to real Chinese life. Whether compounded in Asia for export or in Europe and North America for domestic consumption, these medical commodities were made under western direction, for western tastes, and marketed in accordance with western systems of medical thought (and licensing). Tiger Balm was and is not: it is an Asian product that has succeeded in the western marketplace on its own terms, without reformulation or even rebranding. The same leaping tiger and hexagonal jar, and the same scent, texture, colours, and medicinal contents distinguish the product in its home market in Singapore as in every other of the hundred countries in which it is sold. Moreover, in sharp contrast to, for example, acupuncture in nineteenth-century Britain, Tiger Balm today is recommended and used in each of those countries for the same basic conditions and ailments. So what changes—whether in medical culture, in markets, or in society broadly construed—have enabled Tiger Balm achieve its enviable ubiquity without giving up its Asian identity?

Tiger Balm has always been closely associated with China and with Chinese medicine; however, it has only relatively recently been produced in the People's Republic of China itself. In fact, one of the neatest ironies about the product is that it was created, manufactured, and marketed by sons of the Aw family, Hakka Chinese immigrants to Rangoon (and thence Singapore and Hong Kong) in the late nineteenth century. Whether or not their experience as immigrants endowed the Aw brothers with a particularly well-honed sense of what would appeal to other 'Chinese overseas', they certainly would have been familiar with the institutions, customs, and practices of such communities. And there were Chinese overseas almost everywhere. Waves of Chinese immigrants arrived in the Americas and Australia (and to a lesser extent, Europe) in the second half of the nineteenth century, bringing their own medical culture with them. For the first time, westerners of all classes and backgrounds could see for themselves the medical practices of an equally diverse population of Asians. They gained access to folk as well as elite and scholarly medicine, and were no longer dependent on the reports of observers defending specific economic, political or religious interests. From the *fin de siècle* on, Americans, Europeans, and others—motivated by curiosity, mysticism, fear, loathing, desperation, or simply a taste for novelty—avidly explored in person their new Cathays, their 'Chinatowns'.[3]

Medical professionals did not always welcome the new opportunities for cross-cultural exchange that growing immigrant communities offered to their hosts. Chinese medicine was yet another threat to a profession that was only just beginning to drive out its own indigenous competitors—for instance, homeopathy and mesmerism. In the Australian state of Victoria, burning with gold fever and strangled by epidemic diphtheria in the 1870s, Chinese doctors became the targets of hostile legislation.[4] As the historian and acupuncturist Rey Tiquia has documented, western medical doctors were the principal lobbyists for new regulations intended to exclude the Chinese (as well as competitors from other systems) from practising medicine. Orthodox western practitioners outnumbered Chinese healers by almost ten to one in the 1861 census of Victoria, and were clearly the most prominent healing community. So why did the combination of Chinese healers and intransigent disease produce such a ferocious reaction?

Whether understood as a miasmic disease spread by a filthy and overcrowded environment, or a contagious one spread by infected people, diphtheria was a frightening affront to a profession increasingly convinced of its prowess, and a population desperate to protect its children. In eleven years, Victoria lost 4,574 people to diphtheria; one family lost seven children in twenty days. Orthodox western doctors had little to offer their patients—and they were struggling in a fiercely competitive marketplace against homeopaths, herbalists, and aboriginal healers, as well as the tiny Chinese medical community, and the behemoth of self-medication. When the mainstream press started reporting Chinese success in treating the disease, Western physicians faced not only a loss of market share, but a loss of face: a defeat at the hands of a medical system they saw as the superstitious quackery of an inferior culture. And then, to heap indignity upon injury, their own patients and parliamentarians called upon the orthodox medical profession to validate this foreign remedy through scientific examination.

In 1870, the *Australian Medical Journal* (*AMJ*) printed a letter from a layman, describing the Chinese treatment and enclosing a sample packet of what he referred to as 'John's magic powder' ('John Chinaman' was a common generic sobriquet for the Chinese in the colony). Already, the Chinese treatment—composed of a white powder applied directly onto the infected tissues by blowing through a straw—had spread out from the Chinese poor to the desperate majority community. Burns Malcolm, the *AMJ* correspondent, felt 'compelled to admit, through a world of prejudice' that the powder so administered by a Chinese healer, brought 'great advantage to his clients'. And he urged the editor: 'I hope that you will have the powder examined by some expert . . . so that if there is any real virtue in the powder, we may reap the advantage therefrom and not permit "John" to have a monopoly of the glad tidings.'[5] In 1874, members of Victoria's Parliament responded to such media and voter pressure by debating the appropriateness of a proposed trial of the powders. C. Campbell, Member for Ararat—home to several prominent Chinese practitioners—rubbed salt into open wounds. Not only did he urge the Government to try the Chinese remedy, he justified his request by noting that 'the disease had baffled medical science to a great extent.' Perhaps even worse, he suggested that 'the vast empire of China' could hold at least a few drugs 'which might be of extreme value to this colony'. Campbell even proposed that a Chinese practitioner, Ah Sue, perform the trial according to his usual methods, albeit under medical scrutiny. This was a step too far. The Government protested that subjects for the trial would be hard to find, and instead handed the samples over to the medical profession for experimental use. In other words, while willing to assess the drug for its potential within a western framework, the Government had no interest in sanctioning the system from which it emerged, the practitioners who used it, or their culturally specific patterns of use. Unsurprisingly, perhaps, the orthodox doctors who eventually performed the trial reported the powders inefficacious.[6]

The epidemic continued despite medical and public health efforts, and by November 1874, another trial of the Chinese powders was under way. This time, the drugs were chemically analysed under the auspices of the Medical Society of Victoria and the Technology Museum in Melbourne. Dr John Blair, the surgeon who performed the tests, listed the mundane ingredients of the drugs, and declared them not merely quackish, but actively dangerous as applied by Chinese practitioners (although he performed no clinical tests of either the drugs or the method of application). Dismissing these exotic competitors as 'ignorant pretenders' armed with 'native cunning', he then scolded the press, the public, and the parliamentarians for their credulity in accepting as new and effective drugs that were commonplaces of orthodox medicine, available at any chemist's. He neither raised nor addressed the question of why they were not similarly effective in western practice. This pattern of assuming that medicine from other cultures could and should be assessed by western science—and accepted only when in tune with western scientific models—would become a feature of twentieth- and twenty-first-century responses to cross-cultural medicine.

As the popularity of Chinese medicine during Victoria's diphtheria epidemic illustrates, however, 'scientificity' was no more the sole criterion of nineteenth-century consumers than it is today. Stewart Culin (1858–1929) was not, perhaps, an entirely average Philadelphian. He was, however, a remarkable and curious observer of cross-cultural interactions, living in a country and a historical moment transformed by immigration. A famous and well-travelled ethnographer of games, gambling, and 'secret societies' (and therefore a familiar of the US Chinese communities), Culin turned his attentions to 'The Practice of Medicine by the Chinese in America' in the late 1880s:

Many of the Chinese stores in our American cities keep a supply of Chinese drugs, and all of them sell Chinese proprietary medicines, such as pills to aid digestion, the 'red pills' *Sha hi un* for cholera, catarrh, snuff, and other specifics compounded in the Canton drug shops. These are always neatly packed and labelled, and accompanied with printed directions for their use. But there is often a regular drug business, usually carried on by a separate company, in the stores, and a supply of drugs comprising many, if not all, of those called for in their practice, contained in numerous boxes and drawers on one side of the shop. Here, often, a Chinese doctor, usually some poor and broken down student... has his office.[7]

To extend his studies, Culin became a patient: 'with a desire to learn something of the method of treatment, and obtain some practical knowledge of the Chinese *materia medica*, I recently called upon a doctor connected with one of the principal Chinese stores in Philadelphia, and requested him to prescribe for a cold on the chest from which I was suffering.'

Culin had no axe to grind: he was neither a doctor nor a missionary, nor was he an unwelcome foreign 'guest' on often hostile Chinese soil. Perhaps this is why his first-hand account of Chinese medical practice was so free of the bile and stereotyping characteristic of reportage by Europeans resident in China. His report was broadly positive: 'The practice of medicine among them is comparatively free from superstitious observances.... The doctors show much solicitude about administering any medicine that may cause a fatal result... so that their treatment in general, if not beneficial, does no particular harm to their patients.' Even Culin, however, was taken aback by one feature of Chinese practice: its emphasis on the authority of the pulse. He described the attention with which the Chinese physician took his pulse: 'Then, without inquiring about the symptoms of my complaint, he wrote the prescription...'. Despite almost a century of efforts towards this goal, orthodox western doctors at the end of the nineteenth century still did not assert so absolutely their right to read the sick body without assistance (or interference) from its inhabitant.

Of course, medical exploration and adaptation was only one aspect of western responses to rapidly increasing levels of exposure to other cultures. As in earlier centuries, notions of racial and cultural superiority were pervasive. They continued to be expressed, through fashions like japonisme and chinoiserie, the broader intellectual filter of orientalism, and science-inflected movements like eugenics. Moreover, with mass migration came sometimes-hysterical levels of concern about the importation of disease, vice, and disability (see Figure 21). Combined with widespread popular fear of 'foreign' competition for jobs, these convictions and anxieties could easily erupt into violence against the most visible ethnic groups or enclaves—like the Chinese and Chinatowns. A rash of anti-immigration measures broke out across the destination countries of the West at the end of the nineteenth and beginning of the twentieth centuries, affecting Chinese and Japanese migration particularly harshly.[8] Yet the medical productions of other cultures retained their enduring fascination to consumers; the products, therapies, and cultures in favour changed as quickly as any other fashion, but the idea of a truly different medicine did not lose its appeal. Indeed, a recent study in the United States suggested that not only does the popularity of alternative medicine in general continue to rise, but that it is rising fastest for those therapies that are most distinct from biomedicine.[9]

By the time Chinese and other non-western immigrants were again thronging to northern Europe and North America in the middle of the twentieth century, practitioners of western medicine had finally achieved the levels of authority they had so envied their Chinese counterparts. They were, however, far from demonstrating the 'solicitude' towards their patients that Culin had noted among Chinese doctors. Instead, in the 'Golden Age' of western biomedicine, patients were increasingly depersonalized, their treatment standardized, and their management moved from the home to

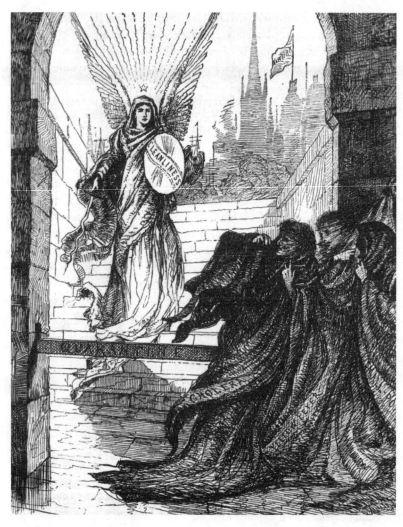

21. 'At the Gates: Our Safety Depends on Official Vigilance', *Harper's Weekly*, New York, 5 September 1885. Cholera, yellow fever, and smallpox, all diseases associated with immigrants and the urban slums in which they were forced by poverty to live, are blocked from entering the Port of New York by a barrier labelled 'Quarantine', and an angel bearing a shield marked 'cleanliness'. This image typifies American attitudes towards immigration as a font of disease, and the new public health policies, shaped by both Sanitarian ideals and germ thinking which emerged from them.

ever-larger and more disorienting hospitals. Medicine had gone 'macho' once again; many of its practitioners dreamed of magic bullet cures and medical firsts. Not all were so sanguine; concern that science was driving a wedge between doctors and their patients was also widespread. Were doctors becoming slaves to the laboratory and abandoning the bedside? In 1926, the famous medical scientist Francis Peabody wrote—in one of the most cited articles of the day

the application of the principles of science to the diagnosis and treatment of disease is only one limited aspect of medical practice. The practice of medicine in the broadest sense is . . . an art, based to an increasing extent on the medical sciences, but comprising much that still remains outside the realm of science . . . [10]

And scientific medicine was also increasingly expensive, whether to the taxpayer, the insurer, or the consumer at the point of delivery. It was institutionally formidable and focused on the cure of acute disease (see Introduction, above). All of these attributes contributed to growing consumer dissatisfaction. So too did events which cast doctors, scientists, and indeed science itself in a morally dubious light: for instance, the active participation of medical scientists in Nazi atrocities, the Tuskegee syphilis experiment (which ran from 1932 to 1972 and left hundreds of African American men and their families suffering from untreated syphilis long after a cure was available), and forced eugenic sterilizations; the role of physics in creating the atom bomb; and of industrial science in pollution and environmental degradation. And then there were the failures of biomedicine, rendered more visible by its many successes: iatrogenic disease, nosocomial infection, antibiotic resistance, thalidomide.

Western consumers were disenchanted by science, and living in societies rapidly transforming around political movements—including feminism, environmentalism, anti-racism, and multiculturalism— dedicated to redressing social imbalances which had often been reinforced by the science of earlier eras. A new cultural focus on individualism, too, went against the grain of biomedical practice and the constantly decreasing time allotted to the doctor–patient encounter within orthodox medicine. This combination of factors sharply stimulated renewed interest in both cross-cultural and alternative medicine. Both were untainted by the whiff of abusive hegemonic power, and both allowed individuals to tailor medical treatment to accord with personal identity, philosophy, and preferences.

One beneficiary of such interest was Tiger Balm. In the early 1960s, in fact, the analgesic balm was one of the best-known symbols of Liverpool's Chinese enclave. In 1961, the Manchester *Guardian* newspaper confidently named this well-established and diverse population—mingling intermarried Irish-Chinese families, a shifting population of sailors, and recent (and significantly for Tiger Balm, primarily Hakka) immigrants from the Hong Kong's New Territories—the 'Tiger Balm community'. The *Guardian*'s reporter observed that, as soon as communication between the two communities became possible, medical exchanges began:

English classes have already made an impression on the Chinese provision shops of Great George Square, where the language barrier used to inhibit access to...the 1,300 herbal medicines ranged round the walls in brown paper parcels. (Even English customers are taking to Tiger Balm, a formidable specific for aches and pains).[11]

Although a major vehicle of transmission, Chinese immigration was not the only route by which Tiger Balm and other non-western medicines found their way into European and North American homes. Burma, Singapore, and Hong Kong were, of course, British colonies when the Aw brothers began to build their Tiger Balm empire. Like their predecessors over the centuries, some British civil servants investigated and took up indigenous medical products for their own use. The older routes of transmission still functioned—but they were far less efficient than the new pathway, leading directly to the markets and pharmacies of European and North American Chinatowns. This process of transmission by consumption continues apace. Today, western consumers can even purchase volumes listing Chinese patent remedies with their uses, ingredients, and histories—and in some cases, including pictures of their packaging, to facilitate their purchase by non-Chinese-speakers in stores predominantly patronized by Chinese-speakers and new immigrants seeking medical home-comforts.[12]

Tiger Balm and other non-western proprietary medicines represent one distinctive aspect of cross-cultural medicine in the late twentieth and early twenty-first century. Although, as preceding chapters have shown, the purely pragmatic acceptance of medical commodities from any culture is not novel, consumers now have direct access to a much wider range of such commodities via large immigrant communities and the services (including internet and mail-order businesses) linked to them. And although medical professionals can and do reinterpret and constrain the medical products of other cultures, consumers need not accept those redefinitions—they can go back to the source themselves, either physically or via the internet and other technologies of global mass communication and translation. Western consumers can now choose to use remedies from anywhere in the world, and to use them as they are deployed in their medical cultures of origin. Nor are Chinatowns or other ethnic communities the only destination for these medical adventurers: Chinese pharmacies offering both herbal and acupuncture treatments are now an everyday feature of British high streets and American strip malls (see Figure 22). Even hikers in the Austrian Tyrol can pick and choose between Ayurvedic therapies. Up to the mid-1990s, many European countries and American states restricted the practice of acupuncture to medical doctors, but these laws were difficult to enforce and are now undergoing reform.

The relaxation of such restrictive legislation should by no means be taken as a sign that alternative and cross-cultural medicine remains an unregulated marketplace, however. The same interdependent processes of regulation and professionalization that dominated the nineteenth-century history of orthodox medicine are now under way in relation to many heterodox disciplines of healing— and for almost exactly the same reasons. The use of complementary, alternative, and cross-cultural medicines has become increasingly mainstream, and these therapeutic modalities are therefore much more visible and more profitable. One major US survey noted that both in 1990 and in 1997, consumers made more visits to 'alternative' practitioners than to all US primary care physicians.[13] No longer condemned *a priori* as 'fringe' or 'quack' healers, heterodox

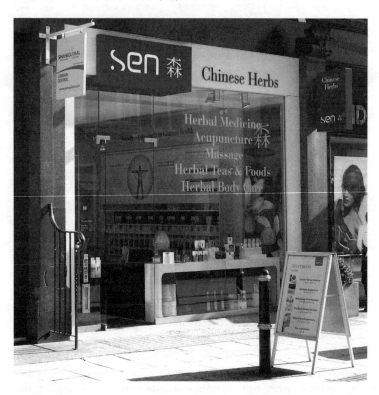

22. 'Sen', Lisa Belsham, London, 2006. This sleek chain of upmarket Chinese medicine salons exemplifies a consumer trend to regard the medicines of other cultures as mainstream 'lifestyle' commodities. It also illustrates the increased visibility of Chinese medicine on the western high street, and the durability of orientalism as a marketing tool for Asian cultural products.

practitioners too are concerned about the effects of competition, widely variable levels of training, and consequent damage to their own and their therapy's reputation. Moreover, such professionals want access to the kinds of resources poured (by governments, insurance companies, industry and charitable foundations) into orthodox medicine: funding for research, for education, and for services to patients less or unable to pay. On the other side of the equation, both cost and consumer demand are encouraging the entities that foot the healthcare bills to look closely at alternative forms of medical provision. The perceived focus of many alternative therapies and modalities on self-healing behaviours sits well with contemporary public health campaigns—and of course, as long as chronic and degenerative illnesses are on the increase and intransigent to biomedical intervention, the cost-effectiveness of alternative therapies for such morbidity will remain appealing. Migraines, depression, back pain, allergies, arthritis, nausea (whether from morning sickness or chemotherapy), addictions, insomnia, and chronic pain: these mundane forms of morbidity have proven unresponsive to biomedical solutions. Meanwhile, the time consumed in repeatedly addressing them biomedically has grown increasingly costly and scarce for patients and practitioners alike.

But governments, especially, are committed to 'evidence-based medicine', and reluctant to spend taxpayers' money on unregulated and unproven procedures. Thus, voices from within the major medical heterodoxies—particularly homeopathy, chiropractic, osteopathy, acupuncture, Ayurveda, 'traditional Chinese medicine', and herbal medicine—are calling for regulation or the legal right to self-regulate. And governments are debating the same issues, while increasing funding for 'scientific' research into the efficacy of heterodox practices (to the disgust of many in the biomedical community). In 1991, Congress mandated the US National Institutes of Health (NIH) to investigate 'unconventional medicine'. The NIH opened its Office of Alternative Medicine in 1992, but budgeted only a paltry $2 million for its operations—0.02 per cent of its budget for research on therapies then used by an estimated 35 per cent of American citizens. After a bitter and protracted battle with Congress, that budget was increased to $50 million in the late 1990s—still less, as one dermatologist pointed out, than was spent on toenail fungus alone.[14] While European governments had a head start in addressing the rising tide of interest in heterodox medicine, they showed little more enthusiasm for funding scientific research into its efficacy or modes of operation. In Britain, the Thatcherite ethos of individual choice and decentralization left many general practitioners managing their own budgets, and with the liberty to purchase alternative medical services if they wished. Many did so, creating a patchwork of data, but few scientifically credible and comparable trials. The response of professional bodies like the British Medical Association and the General Medical Council (GMC) ranged from blandly lukewarm to actively hostile—in testimony to a House of Lords Committee in 1999, the GMC angrily blamed 'a flight from science, fuelled by unbalanced and inaccurate articles in the media and by the unsubstantiated claims from some environmental groups'.[15] And when in late 2006 the British Medicines and Healthcare Regulatory Agency (MHRA) decided to allow homeopathic medicines to make specific therapeutic claims for the first time since 1968, they provoked a furious response from many quarters of the biomedical community. Thirteen different professional bodies, including the Medical Research Council and the Royal Society, protested, and accused the MHRA of yielding to pressure from the alternative medicine industry.

But resistance has proven futile. Where medical professionals have disdained to tread, legislators and public demand have pushed them willy-nilly. The emerging professional bodies of different alternative, complementary, and cross-cultural medicines helped their orthodox brethren accept the inevitable by rendering it more familiar and thus more palatable. With increasing numbers of scientific trials, and westernized forms of non-western medical systems emerging, the essential pragmatism of medical practitioners and consumers alike has facilitated greater acceptance of medical heterodoxies across the board.

A less pragmatic, but even more distinctive, aspect of cross-cultural medicine in the West today is the acceptance not just of medical practices and products, but of medical concepts as well. In a recent study of acupuncture-use in Norway, Gry Sagli observed that both medically and non-medically trained acupuncture practitioners used Chinese concepts when discussing the technique with their colleagues.[16] Asked how acupuncture works, and given free and non-exclusive choice of both biomedical and traditional

Chinese explanations, the majority of practitioners selected as one option the vaguely biomedical 'Acupuncture activates various physiological systems'.[17] But a quarter of all medical doctors, and higher proportions of other practitioners, also accepted and deployed concepts like yin/yang and *qi* to explain the modus operandi of acupuncture. Moreover, members of all groups actually used Chinese medical concepts to explain the technique to colleagues as well as patients; 67 per cent of doctors, for example, used at least one of a range of Chinese concepts (with *qi* and ying/yang being most popular, but also including *zangfu* (organs/bodily networks) and *jingluo* (vessels/meridians/tracts)). Compare this to eighteenth- and nineteenth-century medical responses to Chinese medical theory and body-concepts! And although 75 per cent of doctors saw scientific explanations and models as important to their trust in acupuncture, 45 per cent also found alternative explanations 'reliable'.[18] Again, non-doctors were even more comfortable accepting non-western explanatory systems, with at least 75 per cent relying on Chinese concepts. 57 per cent of these doctors accepted *qi* as referring to a 'real' phenomenon or substance, a rate which rose to 87 per cent among practitioners trained as associated health personnel.[19]

Sagli also discusses another crucial aspect of cross-cultural medicine: education and training in the techniques themselves, and in the theories that underpin them. In the nineteenth century, not only was formal educational provision in acupuncture sporadic, but it was also given exclusively in terms of western explanatory models, which proved both partial and unsatisfying. Some saw acupuncture performed either in China or in the West, but most practitioners learned how to needle simply from reading about it.[20] In the twentieth-first century, there is a wide diversity of routes into acupuncture practice: while some would-be acupuncturists travel to China to participate in either traditional or modern training programmes, others participate in seminars or degree programmes at dedicated western institutions, and many self-educate via the vast and growing literature. Crucially and distinctively, many medical students have the opportunity to study acupuncture and other alternative therapies within orthodox universities or medical schools—60 per cent of US medical schools offered some training on complementary and alternative therapies by 2000, and the University of Exeter in the UK has a chaired professor in Complementary and Alternative Medicine. And as Sagli and others have documented, access to the underlying alternative medical theories plays a substantially greater part in all of these modes of transmission. The concepts and body models underlying cross-cultural, complementary, and alternative medicines also play a significant role in consumer responses to them. As I suggested above, for many users, it is precisely the difference between these systems and biomedicine that lends them their appeal.

A final crucial difference between contemporary and historical waves of interest in both alternative and cross-cultural medicine is signified by the novel category of 'complementary medicine'. Although the terms are often used interchangeably in the media, the modifiers 'complementary' and 'alternative' designate very different relationships to orthodox biomedicine. As I have demonstrated in previous chapters, 'alternative medicine' is practised independently from and often in opposition to medical orthodoxy. Complementary medicine instead is practised as a supplement to orthodox treatments. Instead of confronting biomedicine as an equal, complementary medicine takes either an adjunct or a subordinate role in patient care. Today, most heterodox techniques are practised in both modes—and the practices may be virtually identical in content in either mode. However, the significance and experience of heterodox practices for consumers and providers alike are substantially inflected by a complementary or alternative stance. The distinction—and the degree to which it depends on the trends towards the professionalization, regulation, and integration of heterodox medicine—is evident in a 1997 working document produced for the National Health Service in Scotland:

The word *'complementary'* is preferred to the word *'alternative'* since all systems of medicine have their parts to play in helping to maintain or restore health. It therefore follows that conventional clinicians and complementary practitioners should work together in harmony to achieve this aim ... The term *'complementary practitioner'* is used to refer to a person who has undertaken a recognised training course in a named therapy and has been awarded a qualification by an examining body which meets the identified criteria.[21]

Of course, if a consumer is drawn to a particular practice because it is not orthodox, this normalizing would not necessarily be welcome; as the Report noted, 'if complementary medicine is subsumed within conventional medicine, the opportunity to be "different", and the valued freedom associated with that opportunity could be lost'.[22]

At this point it is appropriate to note, even if this volume cannot discuss at length, the substantial differences between national responses to the rise of alternative, complementary, and cross-cultural medicine. The tone of this Scottish report, and of similar English and Welsh documents, is considerably more positive than that used by Wayne Jonas, then-director of the NIH's Office of Alternative Medicine. In part this may be a matter of audience; in part of timing. By 1997, the Scottish working party had something of a *fait accompli* on its hands; moreover, it was addressing its report to Health Boards already looking for cost-effective solutions, and working with doctors empowered to purchase heterodox medical solutions for their patients. Jonas, writing in 1998 at the end of a turbulent tenure at the Office of Alternative Medicine, was addressing a biomedical audience highly sceptical of alternative medicine and if anything angered by its popular and legislative support in the United States. He was, in fact, still speaking within a climate that had already been much tempered in Europe by greater experience with 'complementary' practice—and the exigencies of national healthcare systems facing an ageing population and searching for creative solutions. And if national styles and responses vary among western nations, what do responses to cross-cultural and alternative medicines look like outside of the West? Are these terms, and the concept of a 'complementary medicine', even meaningful in a non-western context?

With the global dissemination of biomedicine has come a tendency for western policy-makers and institutions to regard indigenous systems of medicine throughout the world as 'alternatives' even in their countries of origin. Thomas Reardon, then-president of the American Medical Association illustrated, but also acknowledged, this perception clearly in 2000: 'Treatments that initially look 'alternative' to Western culture may be part of the medical mainstream in the originating culture. Some estimates suggest that 80% of the world uses "alternative" treatment as their primary means of healthcare while struggling to afford Western medicine.'[23] This was certainly my own experience living in rural Nigeria. Until a nearby town got its first biomedical clinic in the mid-1970s, healing in my village came in two forms: hit-or-miss self-medication with whatever western drugs (often out-of-date, or worse) turned up in the market, or traditional medicine. Even when the clinic opened, its use by villagers depended on the availability of my parents' tiny VW Bug (the only car in the village at that time) and someone to drive it.

Worse, the western tendency to assume the marginality—the 'alternativeness'—of traditional medicine is often paired with a conviction that non-western medical systems are static, or even stagnant. Even medical professionals committed to the study of alternative and cross-cultural medicine fall readily into this trap. Jonas (a committed student of homeopathy as well as director of the NIH's Office of Alternative Medicine) wrote, 'Most alternative medicine systems have been largely unchanged for hundreds or thousands of years.'[24] Of course, such views are unduly simplistic and ethnocentric. In highly populous nations, especially those with low annual incomes and large rural populations, biomedicine remains an 'alternative' to systems of medicine with far better established and denser networks of practitioners, and far lower per capita costs of care. China and India illustrate two different versions of this pattern, particularly outside major urban areas. Post-revolutionary Chinese governments strove to address the medical needs of the vast rural population through a cadre of 'barefoot doctors', trained in basic techniques that drew upon both western and Chinese medical traditions. Post-colonial India began to build a multi-stranded system, supporting Ayurveda and Unani Tibb and homeopathy as well as biomedicine (although biomedicine rapidly absorbed the lion's share of funding).[25] And practitioners of all systems of medicine in each of these pluralist medical cultures have adopted and adapted tools, techniques, and practices from each other: thus acupuncture was dramatically reintroduced to the West through the modern Chinese practice of acupuncture anaesthesia for biomedical surgical operations, while Ayurvedic and Unani healers were quick to adopt stethoscopes, thermometers, and antibiotics.

In fact, at no point—and certainly not over the course of the twentieth century—have indigenous medical systems remained static in the face of biomedicine. From their earliest encounters, medical exchange between systems has been mutual if rarely equal. Although medical 'purists' remain a vocal minority in many non-biomedical systems (including western 'alternative' medicines), responses in general have been more pragmatic. For instance, the adaptive approach to western medical theory, and to 'scientific medicine' visible in Indian responses to the germ-theory controversy (see Chapter 4), has permeated India's thriving medical marketplace since the turn of the twentieth century. One example of this can be found in the early twentieth-century marketing literature of traditional Ayurvedic pharmaceuticals.

Pandit D. Gopalacharlu founded the Madras Ayurvedic Laboratory in the 1890s, to mass-produce Ayurvedic remedies (in fact, at almost the same time that Stewart Culin was setting out to sample the 'neatly packaged' wares of his local Chinese pharmacy).[26] In 1898, he opened the first Ayurvedic dispensary (Ayurvedasramam) in Madras. The dispensary was not only a valuable outlet for the Laboratory's productions, but allowed Gopalacharlu to test them, and reap patient testimonials to their success. These testimonials appeared, alongside the comments of notable Indian and western visitors, in the Madras Ayurvedic Laboratory's mail-order catalogue. In 1901, he extended his facilities even further, opening an Ayurvedic college and later a free Dispensary in which students could gain clinical experience. At each stage, the intimately linked trajectories of his medical and commercial interests and institution building closely parallel those of homeopathy in Europe and North America, and for that matter, the spread of orthodox western medicine in China (where the exigencies of empire did not, as in India, directly determine its form and progress).

By his approach, Gopalacharlu is distinguished as one of an increasing number of modernizers within the Ayurvedic fold, as well as a close observer of western medical trends. A crucial part of the project of modernizing Ayurveda involved incorporating the language and practices of science to restore its lost authority and rescue it from its centuries of 'stagnation'. Thus Gopalacharlu drew attention to his 'laboratory' and asserted frequently that his medicines were 'scientifically prepared'. His elite visitors commented enthusiastically on the progressiveness of his approach. Sir P. N. Krishnamurty, retired dewan of Mysore, testified:

The principal feature which impressed us very favourably in connection with the institution is that on the old Ayurvedic system of medicine is engrafted the modern progressive reform which . . . is brightening this also with the light which we inhabiting the regions of the Rising Sun are now getting only from our happy contact with the receding rays in the far west. . . . Another very useful feature is that to cover the deficiencies of the Hindu system, which are perhaps the evils of a long period of suspense and absence of progressive activity, the Western demonstrative methods of teaching Anatomy and Physiology are adopted.[27]

Even more indicative of the modernizers' tactics is the testimony of Lieutenant-Colonel W. G. King, Sanitary Commissioner to the Government in Madras. King praised Gopalacharlu's 'special knowledge of ancient Hindu medicine' and Sanskrit texts, then noted that, 'at his request I have examined the dispensary at which he works':

I consider the whole arrangements reflect much credit upon himself and the committee concerned . . . Personally I am no believer in 'systems', but consider that science can gather fruit from the tree of experience in whatever soil it grows. There must be drugs that were known and used by ancient Hindus, which, brought to light with the aid of modern methods of phareacology [sic], may prove of great utility. Hence I am glad to see that the institution is conducted in no conservative spirit, but that . . . the teaching of Physiology and Anatomy is recognized as a necessary adjunct of the Ayurvedic students' course.[28]

Narayana Thailum

OR

THE GOUT, RHEUMATISM AND PARALYSIS DESTROYER,

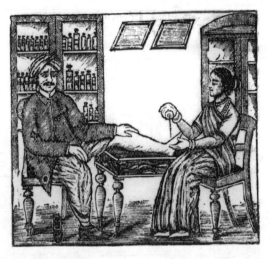

23. 'Narayana Thailum', from Pandit D. Gopalacharlu, *Ayurvedic Medicine prepared ... at the Madras Ayurvedic Laboratory,* 1909. While the image in this catalogue entry shows two traditionally dressed Indians using the advertised salve, they are seated in a room with typically western medicine cabinets and what appear to be western-style diplomas on its walls: a stereotypical western doctor's office. The text uses traditional humoural explanations, but also dwells on scientific preparation of the drug.

So, like Esdaile before him in the nineteenth century, and like proponents of alternative systems in the West today, Gopalacharlu actively sought official attention and scrutiny, as a source of credibility and a sign of official sanction. The images and language Gopalacharlu used to advertise his remedies similarly incorporated both traditional and modern elements (see Figures 23 and 24).

Manasollasini

OR

The Memory Pills.

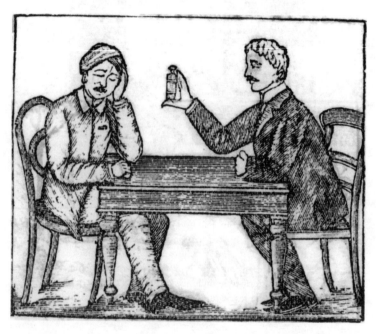

24. 'Manasolasini or The Memory Pills', from Pandit D. Gopalacharlu, *Ayurvedic Medicine prepared . . . at the Madras Ayurvedic Laboratory*, 1909. Here, by contrast, a man in western clothing with light hair is presenting medicine to another man in Indian attire. The text of the advertisement is strikingly similar to that of western patent medicines intended to cure that *fin de siècle* ailment 'neurasthenia', and to address the strains of 'modernity'. But it also used the traditional Ayurvedic language of purification.

Although clearly recognizing the necessity of a response to the challenges of scientific medicine, Ayurvedic practitioners had no desire to erase their heritage, or to replace it with the scientific method. Even the Madras Ayurvedic Laboratory's mail-order catalogue included a lengthy and glowing 'historical sketch of Ayurveda'. And while modernizers worked to assimilate the most desirable aspects of western medicine, they also reached out to defend and raise the status of their own system in the West. Throughout the twentieth century, Ayurvedic practitioners and enthusiasts took every opportunity to present Ayurveda's case before the medical profession. Thus in 1917, for example, the US medical periodical *Medical Times* carried a lengthy transcript of a paper on Ayurvedic medicine presented by Dr Sarat Chandra Ghose to the 1916 Eight Annual Meeting of the American Association of Clinical Research. The paper lauded Ayurveda's glorious past—'Hindu medicine attained a very high level of perfection when the rest of the world was almost in its infancy...long before western medical science came into existence'. It also sketched out Ayurvedic principles, organization, and models of the body; described the discoveries and innovations of Charaka and Susruta—and bemoaned Ayurveda's losses, its 'history of stagnation and decay' caused by religious scruples, invasions, and internal feuding, as losses to medicine as a whole.[29] Articles following this format appeared sporadically in the medical press until the 1970s.

A 1964 *Lancet* editorial exemplifies another way in which information about Ayurveda came to the attention of the medical profession. It also illustrates continuities between orthodox responses to alternative medical systems in the nineteenth century, and to cross-cultural systems in the twentieth century. Titled 'Systems of Medicine', the article opened gloomily: 'Intellectual freedom, like political freedom, is for many people a burden...'. Its author then discussed the emergence, persistence, and gradual 'debasement' of Aristotelian physiological theories. The author argued that, although in the West, these ideas disappeared during the Renaissance, they remained the basis of Unani Tibb and Ayurveda. In faintly scandalized tones, the author noted that Ayurveda has latterly gained increasing importance because it receives so much official encouragement. In well-equipped Ayurvedic hospitals and schools, the students nowadays are smart young men with Westernised general education, and the teachers are far from being the depressed villagers that might be imagined. Indeed, some of these colleges bear the names of distinguished members of our profession who thus lend support to the 'indigenous' medicine of their country.[30]

Not unlike the Orientalists and colonial doctors of the nineteenth century, the author damned with faint praise: 'the hakim employs the highly respectable theory of causality formulated by Aristotle— the theory which in fact most of us use, however outmoded it may be to specialists'; 'Once their fundamental concepts are granted, both indigenous systems are rational enough; they are far from magic and witch-doctoring'. Once again, the advanced state of medicine in ancient India merited mention, as did the pharmacopoeia: 'it is here that much interest still lies. The remedies employed are largely herbal, and apparently they remain crude preparations and hence of variable action ... But they are cheap and thus of great appeal in poor countries.' So far, so much a continuation of the nineteenth- and early twentieth-century western discourse on non-western medicine. The article did note significant changes. The modernization of Ayurveda, its incorporation into the formal institutions of government-sanctioned and sponsored medicine in post-colonial India; and its cost in comparison to the costs of western 'purified drugs' make the system hard to dismiss out-of-hand. But it remained, in the eyes of this observer, a fundamentally dogmatic system—and the author's closing arguments recapitulate with stunning accuracy the late nineteenth-century profession's critiques of alternative medicine:

There is no reason why 'veds' or hakims should not study morbid anatomy, or radiology, not why the facts of physiology or biochemistry should not be acceptable to them. Unfortunately, however, they cannot abandon the hard core of their philosophy—a pattern into which the facts must be made to fit and which must always obtrude into practical deductions. . . . to be chained to any one vehicle for such a purpose is a limitation to intellectual freedom. In science as we understand it, a theory is no more than a useful means of describing a group of phenomena . . . however close to the facts such deductions seem to be, they must never be held to confer a divine mystical truth on the theory . . . Our own tradition . . . is right in bidding us to seek a rational explanation by all relevant means . . .

Unsurprisingly, this analysis of Ayurveda and Unani Tibb provoked a response from an amateur scholar of Ayurveda—however, it focused entirely on refuting the notion that Ayurveda drew upon the Greeks, and on asserting India's status as the birthplace of medicine.[31] In its focus attention to and exclusivity, the response, like the article itself, reiterates the nineteenth-century debates.

Cross-cultural medicine is now receiving the same (often hostile, but often also assimilative) treatment from the medical profession as alternative medicine did in the nineteenth century. Cross-cultural medical practices are also the subject of similar levels of press and public attention. And practitioners of cross-cultural medicine are professionalizing: seeking official regulation; founding bodies to regulate standards and to grant licences; building schools and clinics in which to train succeeding generations of practitioners. Medically trained, traditionally trained, and lay practitioners of techniques like acupuncture and systems like Ayurveda are all competing—and bickering—with each other. And in the midst of it all, consumers may be confused by qualifications, but are spoilt for choice.

Some scholars have argued that medical professionals resist alternative systems of medicine precisely because those systems resist commodification.[32] Yet it is clear that both historically and in contemporary culture, alternative and cross-cultural medical systems have been readily commodified. As Chapters 2 and 4 illustrated, homeopathic medicine threatened its orthodox competitors in part because it could be rendered portable through the use of kits and manuals. Indeed, homeopathy was a successful alternative—and despite its relatively small number of trained practitioners, a powerful threat to orthodox medicine—in part because it had developed two distinctive modes of practice and strands of self-propagation. First, there was the cadre of elite (and elitist) homeopathic practitioners—many converts from the cream of the 'regular' fold—who captured aristocratic and upper-middle-class 'trend-setting' and 'market-shaping' consumers.

Second, and probably more dangerously for the economic survival of the bulk of 'regular' practitioners (general practitioners often practising just at the edge of financial survival in highly competitive urban environments), there were the anti-elitist homeopaths who produced manuals and kits of medicine for lay users at home. Although the homeopathic elite was historically far more visible, it was this submerged body of home users who kept homeopathy alive in the lean times of orthodox medicine's 'Golden Age' in the middle years of the twentieth century. Perhaps it would be more accurate, then, to hypothesize that any practice that resists commodification will struggle to survive in a fiercely competitive medical marketplace—precisely because it is a marketplace, and to some extent, if there is nothing to sell, then there is also nothing to see.

Here a comparison to acupuncture in eighteenth- and nineteenth-century Europe may be particularly revealing. Ten Rhyne, Kaempfer, and subsequent visitors to the Far East noted the fact that in Asia, lay people practised acupuncture on themselves, and that consumer commodities—maps and other tools for locating acu-points, as well as needles, cases and associated devices—were readily and cheaply available. In the eyes of these medical observers, such lay accessibility undermined acupuncture's status as a professional technique, rather than broadened its appeal—it was rarely presented in a favourable light. And when information about acupuncture was transmitted to Europe, largely by doctors in works intended for the use of other doctors, this use of needles to penetrate the surface of the body was in Britain and Europe explicitly cited as a reason to restrict the use of acupuncture to the anatomically knowledgeable. Thus, the practice of acupuncture in the West was to be limited to the regularly trained, and particularly surgeons—who would use their exclusive knowledge of anatomy, rather than any commercially available and unduly accessible maps or models, to guide their needling. Knowledge of it meanwhile was also limited—first by language (early accounts like Ten Rhyne's were published in Latin); then by access to medical periodicals and monographs, or proximity to either the scattered centres of acupuncture use or an interested individual practitioner.

But today, cross-cultural medicine is far more accessible to a far wider audience; in this, it is more like the highly popular and well-known alternative medicine of the nineteenth century. In part because of the vastly expanded wealth of accessible information about cultures and societies worldwide, more people can gain access to a variety of medical systems and purchase the medical productions of a global marketplace. Descriptions of non-western models of the body, and understandings of health and disease are available in a plethora of different formats, from web ads, to scholarly and other specialist journals, to TV documentaries. Perhaps most importantly of all, both immigration and the emergence of the leisure travel industry has meant that more people have the chance to see medicine from other cultures in practice, on the ground, with their own eyes—to judge for themselves if *qi* or *prana* are more or less credible, comprehensible, and intellectually attractive than neurotransmitters or the Krebs cycle.

FURTHER READING

As well as the primary sources mentioned in the endnotes for each chapter, I drew upon the work of many other scholars in writing this book, both directly (as cited in the endnotes, again) and indirectly. Some readers may wish to delve further into the historical periods and problems this book explores. For them, I recommend the following texts as preliminary starting points. I've organized them by chapter, and note which themes are treated in each.

INTRODUCTION: 'RIVAL SYSTEMS OF MEDICINE'?

Because this chapter addresses so many broad themes, and such a wide geographical and temporal span, I can mention only a fraction of the rich scholarship out there for readers to enjoy. I've chosen to focus on historical (rather than practical or medical) texts which are widely available, and, most importantly, easily and pleasurably readable.

Few texts survey all three of the medical systems I've treated. Of these, probably only Roy Porter, *The Greatest Benefit to Mankind: A Medical History of Humanity from Antiquity to the Present* (New York: W. W. Norton and Co., 1999) fits all of my criteria. An alternative to Porter's broad canvas can be found in Don Bates (ed.), *Knowledge and the Scholarly Traditions* (Cambridge: Cambridge University Press, 1995). A collection of scholarly, but imminently readable, essays, this volume opens windows onto moments in Chinese, Galenic western, and Ayurvedic medicine.

An entirely different approach can be seen in Kenneth Kiple (ed.), *The Cambridge World History of Human Disease* (Cambridge: Cambridge University Press, 1993), and its little brother, Kenneth Kiple (ed.), *The Cambridge Historical Dictionary of Disease* (Cambridge: Cambridge University Press, 2003). These two volumes are inordinately valuable resources, sketching out and defining (the former in depth, the latter concisely) the subject matter at the heart of the history of medicine: the diseases and conditions themselves. It is to these books that readers can turn in search of an explanation of 'relapsing fever' or 'dropsy', or to learn where in the world such conditions might be prevalent—and in the former, they will find fairly straightforward descriptions of the major medical systems of the world.

Western Medicine

Both Mark Harrison, *Disease and the Modern World: 1500 to the Present Day* (Cambridge: Polity Press, 2004) and David Wooton, *Bad Medicine: Doctors Doing Harm since Hippocrates* (Oxford: Oxford University Press, 2006) are polemical texts covering wide swathes of time and space—this makes them both much more fun to read than the run of the mill surveys of the history of western medicine. Harrison joins a lively and empathetic discussion of the emergence of 'modern' medical practices and institutions with some wonderfully clear summations of the different historical approaches which have been taken towards these developments. Wooton on the other hand tackles a long-standing problem in the history of medicine: why did people believe in medical practices, theories, and claims that to our eyes look manifestly absurd—and why do historians of medicine (and I include myself here) resist narratives of 'progress'? Galloping from Hippocrates to heart attacks and lung cancer, he tracks the failure of new knowledge to displace the old in medicine. Of course, polemics are by their nature biased: read these two with pleasure, but also with a few grains of salt. For a more neutral account, see Roy Porter's *Blood and Guts: A Short History of Medicine* (London: Penguin Books, 2002), a breezily concise treatment of the historical timespan. Lawrence Conrad, Michael Neve, Vivian Nutton, Roy Porter, and Andrew Wear, *The Western Medical Tradition 800 BC to AD 1800* (Cambridge: Cambridge University Press, 1995) offers additional detail—and covers classical, medieval, and Arabic medicine in considerably more detail than I have done here. Bill Bynum's *Science and the Practice of Medicine in the Nineteenth Century* (Cambridge: Cambridge University Press, 1994) is the classic slim account of the period and 'the rise of science'. Those specifically interested in medicine in the US context should dip into the excellent collection edited by Judith Walzer Leavitt and Ronald L. Numbers, *Sickness and Health in America* (Madison: University of Wisconsin Press, various editions). The obvious (and rewarding) choice for those interested in medicine since the nineteenth century is Roger Cooter and John Pickstone's edited collection, *Medicine in the Twentieth Century* (Amsterdam: Harwood Academic Publishers, 2000).

Asian Medicine

Charles Leslie and Allan Young (eds.), in *Paths to Asian Medical Knowledge* (Oxford: University of California Press, 1992) have brought together an interesting and interdisciplinary collection assessing Asian medicine broadly construed and in a number of periods. Paul Unschuld, *Medicine in China: A History of Ideas* (Berkeley and Los Angeles: University of California Press, 1985) is a classic and elegantly readable account of Chinese medicine, one that sets its historical development into social and political context—yet doesn't skimp on the actual texts. Shigehisa Kuriyama, *The Expressiveness of the Body: And the Divergence of Greek and Chinese Medicine* (New York: Zone Book, 1999) explores the different ways in which Greek and Chinese healers and philosophers selected and interpreted the available observational and experiential data about the human body. To debunk notions that Chinese medicine has remained static, one has only to open Elisabeth Hsu's edited collection *Innovation in Chinese Medicine* (Cambridge: Cambridge University Press, 2001). Nathan Sivin, *Traditional Medicine in Contemporary China* (Ann Arbor: University of Michigan Press, 1987) does what it says on the label, and does it well. J. Van Alphen and A. Aris (eds.), *Oriental Medicine: An Illustrated Guide to the Asian Arts of Healing* (London: Serindia Publications, 1995), violates one of my principal criteria, in not being particularly easy to find. Its editors offer functional discussions of major aspects of Asian medicine, both historical and contemporary. The real wealth of this text, however, is in its lavish illustrations. Dominik Wujastyk, *Sanskrit Medical Writings* (New Delhi: Penguin, 1998) offers both fresh translations of sometimes arcane texts, and a clear and useful introduction to his sources and the tradition of which they are a part. In *Fluent Bodies: Ayurvedic Remedies for Postcolonial Imbalance* (London: Duke University Press, 2002), Jean Langford looks at the modernization of Ayurveda from a postcolonial perspective, and offers great insights into the intercalation of biomedical and Ayurvedic practices. Although at times theoretically dense, this book is worth the effort.

1. 'WHAT IS THIS BURNING?'

Everyone, but everyone, should read Michael Adas, *Machines as the Measure of Men: Science, Technology, and Ideologies of Western Dominance* (Ithaca: Cornell University Press, 1989)—a fantastic study of western responses to and evaluations of the non-western world from the Age of Exploration to the twentieth century. Intellectually, it is a crucial source and inspiration for global approaches to history, and incidentally my own work—though my examples are of course drawn from medicine, rather than science and technology. And it's a great, if sometimes challenging, read.

To get a vivid picture of the experience of patients in the seventeenth-century European medical world, look at Lucinda McCray

Beier, *Sufferers and Healers: The Experience of Illness in Seventeenth-Century England*. The essays in Roger French and Andrew Wear (eds.), *The Medical Revolution of the Seventeenth Century* (Cambridge: Cambridge University Press, 1989) offer background on the changes which began to reshape western attitudes to non-western and to scholastic medicine.

2. HEALTH AND 'THE NEW SCIENCE'

As the endnotes suggested, three sources are vital for this chapter: Martin Kaufman, *Homeopathy in America* (Baltimore: Johns Hopkins Press, 1971); Phillip Nicholls, *Homoeopathy and the Medical Profession* (London: Croom Helm, 1988); and Alison Winter, *Mesmerized: Powers of Mind in Victorian Britain* (Chicago: University of Chicago Press, 1998). The first two not only delineate the professional chaos, competition, and eventually crises provoked by the advent of homeopathy, but are enriched, through extensive quotations, by the voices of the period in the US and UK respectively. Alison Winter does the same for the subject of mesmerism, and in addition compellingly connects the medical technique with its scientific and popular forms, and the broader social context—and it is indeed astonishingly broad. For another lively read, and another perspective on the interplay between popular and expert understandings of the natural world, see Harriet Ritvo, *The Animal Estate: The English and Other Creatures in Victorian England* (Cambridge, Mass.: Harvard University Press, 1987).

On the subject of quackery, see Roy Porter, *Quacks: Fakers and Charlatans in English Medicine* (Stroud: Tempus Publishing 2000); Porter brings to vivid—and sometimes squalid, scandalous, and grasping—life the medical marketplace in all its eighteenth-century glory. Moreover, he illustrates (and this text is indeed lavishly illustrated) exactly why 'alternative medicine' had no place in it. Dorothy Porter and Roy Porter, *Patient's Progress: Doctors and Doctoring in Eighteenth Century England* (Cambridge: Polity Press, 1989) details the doctor–patient relationship with equal élan and enthusiasm.

Meanwhile, on Enlightenment science, readers can turn to William Clark, Jam Golinski, and Simon Schaffer (eds.), *The Sciences in Enlightened Europe* (Chicago: University of Chicago Press, 1999), a broad and rich collection of excellent essays, particularly for the exact sciences. Nick Jardine, Jim Secord, and Emma Spary, *Cultures of Natural History* (Cambridge: Cambridge University Press, 1996) is equally rich, and beautifully written. Its emphasis on emerging approaches to understanding the natural world makes it particularly accessible and interesting.

3. 'THE CHINESE HAVE A GREAT DEAL OF WIT'

For background on the Scientific Revolution, have a look at Steven Shapin, *The Scientific Revolution* (Chicago: University of Chicago Press, 1998), and Charles Webster's *The Great Instauration* 2nd edn. (Oxford: Peter Lang, 2002). While the former offers an overview, the latter looks closely at the case of England, and particularly at the interplay between the Scientific and the Cromwellian revolutions. A huge volume, it demands the reader's attention—but more than rewards its readers' efforts. Steve Shapin and Simon Schaffer's *The Leviathan and the Air Pump* (Princeton: Princeton University Press, 1989) is likewise based in England—and will swiftly dispel any notions readers may have that scientific discovery is an apolitical or a 'natural' process. Peter Gay's *The Enlightenment: An Interpretation* (New York: W. W. Norton, 1996) is a classic. It can be usefully read with either of the texts listed above for Enlightenment science, as can Roy Porter, *The Enlightenment* (Basingstoke: Palgrave, 2001). Porter's manifest delight in his period, and his determination to portray Britain's unique contributions to the Enlightenment enterprise, enliven this book.

Readings more specific to this chapter can be found in Robert A. Bickers (ed.), *Ritual and Diplomacy: The Macartney Mission to China, 1792–1794* (London: Wellsweep/British Association for Chinese Studies, 1993); Stanley J. Reiser, *Medicine and the Reign of Technology* (Cambridge: Cambridge University Press, 1978)—the classic and as yet unsuperseded text on medicine and technology—and Lucille Brockway, *Science and Colonial Expansion: The Role of the British Royal Botanic Gardens* (New York: Academic Press, 1979). To get a flavour of medical culture and medical politics in the early nineteenth century, readers might want to look at Adrian Desmond, *The Politics of Evolution: Morphology, Medicine and Reform in Radical London* (Chicago: University of Chicago Press, 1989). Focused on Britain, it is packed with wonderful character sketches, and insight. It is, however, not for the faint-hearted or the squeamish. The classic historical work on acupuncture is Gwei Lu and Joseph Needham, *Celestial Lancets: A History and Rationale of Acupuncture and Moxa* (Cambridge: Cambridge University Press, 1980). Readers who wish to explore in greater detail the historical transmission of acupuncture to the West, and specifically to Britain may wish to read an earlier (and more academic) work of my own: Roberta Bivins, *Acupuncture, Expertise and Cross-Cultural Medicine* (Basingstoke: Palgrave, 2000). For further readings on homeopathy see, above, Chapter 2.

4. 'WITH OUR WESTERN BRETHREN, THE CASE SEEMS TO BE QUITE DIFFERENT'

Edward Said, *Orientalism: Western Conceptions of the Orient* (New York: Pantheon Books, 1978) is a foundation text in studies of imperialism and hegemony—and good, if challenging and polemical, reading. The litera-ture on colonial medicine is growing rapidly. This chapter looks first to David Arnold, *Colonizing the Body: State Medicine and Epidemic Diseases in Nineteenth Century India* (Berkeley and Los Angeles: University of California Press, 1993). For an earlier period, see M. N. Pearson, 'First Contacts between Indian and European Medical Systems: Goa in the Sixteenth Century', in David Arnold (ed.), *Warm Climates and Western Medicine* (Amsterdam: Rodopi, 1996), 20–41; Waltraud Ernst has edited a useful collection of scholarly essays which cover a number of relevant topics in *Plural Medicine: Tradition and Modernity, 1800–2000* (London: Routledge, 2002). Alterative approaches to mesmerism in India can be found in Alison Winter, *Mezmerized*, 187–212, and Waltraud Ernst, 'Colonial Psychiatry, Magic and Religion: The Case of Mesmerism in British India', *History of Psychiatry*, 15/1 (2004), 57–71. Alternative perspectives on the movement of medical knowledge and expertise from one culture to another are available in Andrew Cunningham and Bridie Andrews (eds.), *Western Medicine as Contested Knowledge: Studies in Imperi-alism* (Manchester: Manchester University Press, 1997). Readers interested in smallpox should see Sanjoy Battacharya, Mark Harrison, and Michael Worboys, *Fractured States: Smallpox, Public Health, and Vaccination Policy in British India, 1800–1947* (Hyderabad: Orient Longman, 2005)

For recent scholarship on germ theory, see Michael Worboys, *Spreading Germs: Disease Theories and Medical Practice in Britain, 1865–1900* (Cam-bridge: Cambridge University Press, 2000). Nancy Tomes, *Gospel of Germs: Men, Women and the Microbe in American Life* (Cambridge, Mass.: Harvard Univeristy Press, 1998) delightfully demonstrates the power of germ-thinking in reshaping (American) life in the late nineteenth and early twentieth centuries.

CONCLUSION: PRAGMATISM, PLURALISM, AND THE (IM)PATIENT-CONSUMER

There are relatively few book-length historical treatments of alternative, cross-cultural, or complementary medicine in the twentieth century. One of the few, Robert Jütte, Motzi Eklöf, and Marie C. Nelson (eds.), *His-torical Aspects of Unconventional Medicine: Approaches, Concepts, Case Studies*

(Sheffield, European Association for the History of Medicine and Health Publications, 2001), presents some highly relevant material. Hans Baer, *Biomedicine and Alternative Healing Systems in America: Issues of Class, Race, Ethnicity, and Gender* (Madison: University of Wisconsin Press, 2001) also tackles all three areas—though Baer is an anthropologist rather than a historian. Ursula Sharma, *Complementary Medicine Today: Patients and Practitioners*, rev. edn. (London: Routledge, 1995) offers valuable data from a sociological perspective. I've looked in more depth at acupuncture in the twentieth-century context in 'Acupuncture and Innovation: "New Age" Medicine in the NHS', in Jennifer Stanton (ed.), *Innovations in Health and Medicine* (London: Routledge, 2002), 84–105. Ken Zysk has made a similar examination of Ayurveda in 'New Age Ayurveda or What happens to Indian medicine when it comes to America', *Traditional South Asian Medicine*, 6 (2001), 10–26.

On the other hand, many texts look at the issues from a medical and assessment perspective. Phil Fontanarosa (ed.), *Alternative Medicine: An Objective Assessment* (Chicago: American Medical Association, 2000); Charles Vincent and Adrian Furnham, *Complementary Medicine: A Research Perspective* (Chichester, John Wiley and Sons, 1997) are just two of the options here in this crowded field.

Readers might also want to look at the interplay of medicine and immigration. A classic and very approachable text is Alan Kraut, *Silent Travellers: Germs, Genes and the 'Immigrant Menace'* (Baltimore: Johns Hopkins University Press, 1994). I also recommend Amy Fairchild, *Science at the Borders: Immigrant Medical Inspection and the Shaping of the Modern Industrial Labor Force* (Baltimore: Johns Hopkins University Press, 2003); Nayan Shah, *Contagious Divides: Epidemics and Race in San Francisco's Chinatown* (Berkeley and Los Angeles: University of California Press, 2001); and Alexandra Minna Stern, *Eugenic Nation: Faults and Frontiers of Better Breeding in Modern America* (Berkeley and Los Angeles: University of California Press, 2005). All of these volumes address immigration in the United States. For wider geographical coverage, see Lara Marks and Michael Worboys (eds.), *Migrants, Minorities and Health* (London: Routledge, 1997).

But perhaps best, as a way to explore the sensation of being in a different medical culture, is a volume looking at the experience of cross-cultural medicine from the perspective of recent migrants to the West: one such account, and one of the most moving books I've read is Anne Fadiman's *The Spirit Catches You and You Fall Down* (New York: Noonday Press, 1998), an intimate study of the medicalized life and death of Lia Lee, daughter of a family of Hmong refugees in California's Central Valley. Readers who are really hooked after reading Fadiman can go on to Lillian Faderman's *I Begin My Life All Over Again: The Hmong and the American Immigrant Experience* (Boston: Beacon Press, 1998) which incorporates Hmong immigrants' accounts of every aspect of their new and old lives—and the clash between them.

Finally, another wonderful way to access medical knowledge is through its visual heritage. For this, two good starting points are the US National Library of Medicine's many visual resources and online exhibitions, and the iconographic collections of the Wellcome Library in London. See the National Library of Medicine's History homepage at http://www.nlm.nih.gov/hmd/ihm, and the Wellcome Library's collections at http://images.wellcome.ac.uk.

NOTES

INTRODUCTION: 'RIVAL SYSTEMS OF MEDICINE'?

1. Both terms, 'heterodox' and 'alternative', proclaim the fact that these medical practices and theories are not part of, and may directly contradict, the accepted or 'orthodox' system of medical knowledge and practices.

2. This and subsequent quotations are taken from 'Spirit of the British Periodicals', *Journal of the Calcutta Medical and Physical Society*, 1 (1 Jan. 1837), 66.

3. The term 'biomedicine' is particularly useful as an indicator of the distinctive cultural and intellectual ties between the biological sciences and contemporary medical practice and knowledge in the twentieth century, and the degree to which medical authority now depends on its claims to scientificity. In other periods, terms including 'humoural medicine', 'scholastic medicine', and 'regular medicine' will more accurately describe the dominant medical system of the day.

4. See Jonathan Swift, *Gulliver's Travels* (1726). Available in many editions, and also online at http://www.jaffebros.com/lee/gulliver/index.html

5. Jonathan Swift, 'A Voyage to Laputa', in *The Basic Writings of Jonathan Swift* (New York: Modern Classics Library Edition, 2002), 510.

6. Ibid. 522.

7. Jonathan Swift, 'A Further Account of Glubdubdrib: Antient and Modern History corrected', in *The Basic Writings of Jonathan Swift*, op. cit., 540–1.

8. Swift, 'A Voyage to Laputa', 522.

9. J. V. Pickstone, 'Establishment and Dissent in Nineteenth Century Medicine: An Exploration of Some Correspondences and Connections between Religious and Medical Belief-Systems in Early Industrial England', in W. J. Shiels (ed.), *Studies in Church History*, xix (Oxford: Oxford University Press, 1992), 165–89, at 171.

10. Geoffrey Chaucer, *Canterbury Tales,* available in many editions, including *The Works of Geoffrey Chaucer*, ed. F. N. Robinson (London: Oxford University Press, 1957) and online at http://www.bl.uk/treasures/caxton/homepage.html.

11. Margaret Trawick, 'Death and Nurturance in Indian Systems of Healing', in Charles Leslie and Allan Young (eds.), *Paths to Asian Medical Knowledge* (Berkeley and Los Angeles: University of California Press, 1992), 129–59.

12. The traditional literature of Indian medicine is almost entirely written in the ancient language Sanskrit. Throughout this discussion of Indian medicine, I will be using Dominik Wujastyk's new translations of the Sanskrit terms. For extended translations of Sanskrit texts, see Wujastyk, *Sanskrit Medical Writings* (New Delhi: Penguin, 1998); and his essay, 'Medicine in India', in J. Van Alphen and A. Aris (eds.), *Oriental Medicine: An Illustrated Guide to the Asian Arts of Healing* (London: Serindia Publications, 1995), 19–37.

13. Paul Unschuld, *Medicine in China: A History of Ideas* (Berkeley and Los Angeles: University of California Press, 1985) which I heartily recommend to curious readers.

14. Wang Xuanjie and John Moffett, *Traditional Chinese Therapeutic Exercises: Standing Pole* (Beijing: Foreign Languages Press, 1994).

15. Sir John Floyer, *The Physician's Pulse-Watch; Or, An Essay to Explain the Old Art of* FEELING *the* PULSE, *and to Improve it by the Help of a Pulse-Watch* (London: Samuel Smith and Benjamin Walford, 1701), 229.

16. Ibid. 230–1.

17. Ibid. 'Preface', 3.

18. Ibid. 429.

19. Quoted in Roy Porter, *Greatest Benefit to Mankind: A Medical History of Humanity* (New York: W. W. Norton and Co., 1999), 248.

CHAPTER 1: 'WHAT IS THIS BURNING?'

1. Hermann Busschof, *Two Treatises, The One Medical, Of the Gout, and its Nature . . . With a New Way of Discharging the Same; The Other, Partly Chirurgical, Partly Medical; . . . English'd Out of the Dutch by a Careful Hand* (London: Moses Pitt, 1676), This and all subsequent Busschof quotations are drawn from this volume.

2. Cited in n. 1, above.

3. Ibid., 108.

4. Cautery, in its European form, used either actual fire, red hot metal, or caustic chemicals to burn the flesh, sometimes down to the bone. It was used primarily in surgery (for instance, to control blood loss).

5. Busschof, *Two Treatises,* 104–5.

6. John Comrie (ed.), *Selected Works of Thomas Sydenham MD with a Short Biography and Explanatory Notes* (London: John Bale, Sons, and Danielsson, 1922), 67.

7. John Hill, *The Management of the Gout, with the Virtues of Burdock Root, First Us'd in the Author's Own Case, and Since in Many Other Successful Instances*, 8th edn. (London: R. Baldwin, 1771), 15.

8. Sir William Temple, *Miscellanea: By a Person of Honour* (London: Edward Gellibrand, 1680), 207.

9. Comrie (ed.), *Selected Works of Sydenham*, 78–9.

10. Thomas Sydenham, 'A Treatise on Gout, and Dropsy', in *The Works of Thomas Sydenham*, ii, trans. R. G. Latham (London: Sydenham Society, 1850), 161. It is worth noting that gout, although now treatable, remains incurable.

11. T. Garlick, *An Essay on the Gout* (London: T. Warner, 1729), pp. i–ii.

12. Temple, *Miscellanea*, 194.

13. Ibid. 195–6.

14. Ibid. 197–8.

15. Ibid. 189–90.

16. Ibid. 205.

17. Ibid. 204–5.

18. Ibid. 215.

19. Ibid. 217.

20. Quoted in Roy Porter and G. S. Rousseau, *Gout: The Patrician Malady* (London: Yale University Press, 1998), 127.

21. Busschof, *Two Treatises*, 5–6.

22. See also Porter and Rousseau, *Gout*.

23. Sir John Floyer, *The Physician's Pulse-Watch*, 337. Temple's account of his 'experiment' with moxabustion highlights the role of these factors in piquing his interest in an outlandish (literally) medical practice. It also demonstrates the importance of personal networks in the transmission of cross-cultural medical practices and expertise. Temple initially heard about moxabustion from a friend whom he called Monsieur Zulichem— identified by scholars as the diplomat Constantijn Huygens (father of the physicist Christiaan Huygens), who corresponded with the Secretary of the Royal Society. Huygens himself had learned of moxabustion 'by the Relation of several who had seen and tried it in the *Indies*, but particularly by an ingenious little Book'—Busschof's book on the subject. From Huygens, Temple borrowed Busschof's text, and was persuaded by it to send his personal physician to Utrecht (where Busschof's son resided) for moxa and further instruction.

24. Temple, *Miscellanea*, 207.

25. Thomas Peregrine Courtenay, *Memoirs of the Life, Works, and Correspondence of Sir William Temple, Bart*, ii (London: Longman, Beer, Orme, Brown, Green, & Longman. 1836), 104. Rafflesia are a genus of parasitic plants endemic to South-East Asia. They produce the world's largest blossoms, including several carrion-scented varieties.

26. Temple, *Miscellanea*, 211.

27. Busschof, *Two Treatises*, 104–5.

28. Ibid. 105.

29. Temple, *Miscellanea*, 211–12.

30. Busschof, *Two Treatises*, 109. It may be worth noting here that seven-teenth- and eighteenth-century orthography was far from consistent in relation to names. Thus the name I have written as 'Wilhem Ten Rhyne' in this text might also appear as 'William de Ryne', 'Willem Ten Rhijne', and, as above, 'Wilhelmus de Ryne'. Similarly, I have used 'Busschof' but the same person was also called 'Busschofius', 'Busschoff', and, at least once, 'Bisschof'.

31. Robert Carrubba and John Z. Bowers, 'The Western World's First Detailed Treatise on Acupuncture: Willem Ten Rhijne's De Acupunctura', *Journal of the History of Medicine and Allied Sciences*, 29/4 (1974), 377–8. Ten Rhyne refers to Iwanga Sokaa and Motogi Shodayu respectively. Ten Rhyne described the questions as 'Bothersome trifles, to be sure.' Carrubba and Bowers note that Ten Rhyne's answers to some 150 questions like ' "Why do you feel only the left pulse?" ' and ' "How do you differentiate the Yang-type carbuncle and the Yin-type carbuncle?" ' were later published in *Zen-seishi-Tsuiwa*, vol. i bk. 2 (1680), p. 372.

32. Carrubba and Bowers, 'De Acupunctura', 377–8.

33. Ibid. 375.

34. Engelbert Kaempfer, *A History of Japan*, ii (London, 1728), App. p. 39.

35. Ibid.

36. Ibid. 40.

37. Ibid.

38. Ibid. 42.

39. Ibid. 210.

40. Kaempfer also saw environmental conditions as important in the oper-ation. He specifically cautioned Europeans against expecting the same stellar successes from moxabustion in chilly Europe that it produced in sultry Asia. Indeed, he noted that one disappointed European physician had sent a letter of complaint to a prominent Batavia-based physician and moxabustion proponent.

41. Kaempfer, *A History of Japan*, 43.

42. 'An Account of a Book, viz. Wilhelmi ten Ryne M.D. &c. . . . I. dissertatio de Arthritide. 2. Mantissa Schematica: 3. de Acupunctura. . . . Londini in 8vo 1683'. *Philosophical Transactions*, 13 (1683), 222–35, at 222.

43. Kaempfer, *A History of Japan*, 30.

44. Ibid. 32.

45. Ibid. 32.
46. Baron D. J. Larrey, *On the Use of Moxa as a Therapeutical Agent*, trans. Robely Dunglison (London: Thomas and George Underwood 1822), 8. Larrey was surgeon-in-chief to the Hôpital de la Garde Royale, an inspector-general in the Service of Military Health, and Premier-Surgeon to the Grande Armée during Bonaparte's campaigns in Russia, Saxony, and France in 1812–14.

CHAPTER 2: HEALTH AND 'THE NEW SCIENCE'

1. Principal secondary sources for this chapter: Martin Kaufman, *Homeopathy in America* (Baltimore: Johns Hopkins Press, 1971); Phillip Nicholls, *Homoeopathy and the Medical Profession* (London: Croom Helm, 1988); Alison Winter, *Mesmerized: Powers of Mind in Victorian Britain* (Chicago: University of Chicago Press, 1998).
2. Harriet Martineau, *Letters on Mesmerism* (London: Edward Moxton, 1845), pp. vi–vii.
3. Winter, *Mesmerized*, 156.
4. Martineau, *Letters*, pp. vii–viii.
5. James Esdaile, *Mesmerism in India, and its Practical Application in Surgery and Medicine*, ed. David Esdaile (London: Longman, Brown, Green and Longmans, 1846), pp. xviii–xix.
6. Samuel Hahnemann, *Organon of Medicine: A New Translation*, trans. Jost Kunzu, Alain Naudé, and Peter Pendleton (London: Victor Gollancz, 1986), 188. Unless otherwise noted, all quotations from Hahnemann are from this translation of Hahnemann's sixth (and last) revised edition of his *Organon*, completed in 1842, just before his death.
7. Ibid. 15.
8. e.g. the flu might be said to progress through headaches, to swollen glands and body aches, to fever and nausea, to the breaking of the fever, to recuperation.
9. Hahnemann, *Organon*, 25.
10. Trans. Elizabeth Danciger, in *The Emergence of Homeopathy: Alchemy into Medicine* (London: Century Paperbacks, 1987).
11. Trans. Edward Hamlyn, *The Healing Art of Homeopathy* (Chicago: Keats Publishing, 1981), 19.
12. Trans. Danciger, *Emergence of Homeopathy*.
13. Trans. Hamlyn, *Healing Art*, 37–8.
14. Hahnemann, *Organon*, 86.
15. 'News. From "The Times." A newspaper printed in Alexandria, dated in December', *Medical Repository*, 3 (1800), 311–12, quoted in John

Harley Warner and Janet Tighe, *Major Problems in the History of American Medicine and Public Health* (New York: Houghton Mifflin, 2001), 57–8. For a full and gory description of the full extent of 'heroic medicine' see Kaufman, *Homeopathy in America*, esp. ch. 1.

16. Emily Mason to Catherine Mason Rowland, 4 Nov. 1840, quoted in Kaufman, *Homeopathy in America*, 12.

17. As we will see in Chapter 4, homeopathy proved equally adaptable to the political, cultural, and medical climate of colonial India/the Raj.

18. 'American vs. European Medical Science again', *Medical Record*, 4 (1869), 183.

19. *United States Magazine and Democratic Review*, 22 (May 1848), 418, quoted in Kaufman, *Homeopathy in America*, 30.

20. 'Mr. Kingdon on Homeopathy', *Journal of the Calcutta Medical and Physical Society*, 1 (1 July 1837), 404.

21. Sir John Forbes, *Of Nature and Art in the Cure of Disease*, 2nd edn. (London: John Churchill, 1858), 162–3, cited in Nicholls, *Homoeopathy*, 165.

22. Forbes, *Of Nature and Art*, 162–3, cited ibid. 165–6.

23. Forbes, *Of Nature and Art*, 162–3, cited ibid. 166.

24. R. E. Dudgeon, *Hahnemann, The Founder of Scientific Therapeutics* (London: E. Gould and Sons, 1882), 23–4, cited ibid. 169.

25. R. E. Dudgeon, *The Influence of Homeopathy*, 32–3 *on General Medical Practice since the Death of Hahnemann* (London: Turner & Co., 1874), cited ibid.

26. James Esdaile, *The Introduction of Mesmerism (with the Sanction of the Government) into the Public Hospitals of India* (London: W. Kent and Co., 1856), 10.

27. This and immediately succeeding quotations from James Esdaile, *The Introduction of Mesmerism, as an Anaesthetic and Curative Agent into the Hospitals of India* (Perth: Dewar and Son, 1852), 9.

28. Joseph Longshore, in a manuscript biography of his physician wife, Hannah Longshore. Quoted in Regina Morantz-Sanchez, *Sympathy and Science: Women Physicians in American Medicine* (New York: Oxford University Press, 1985), 59.

29. James John Garth Wilkinson, *War, Cholera, and the Ministry of Health, and Appeal To Sir Benjamin Hall and the British People* (New York: William Radde, and Fowler & Wells, 1855). Wilkinson was a regular MD, and author of another (rather curiously titled) work, *The Human Body and its Relation to Man*.

30. Morantz Sanchez, in *Sympathy and Science*, 5 and *passim*, has discussed these themes in great depth.

31. Wilkinson, *War*, 54.

32. Ibid, 53.

33. Anne Taylor Kirschmann, 'Adding Women to the Ranks, 1860–1890: A New View with a Homeopathic Lens', *Bulletin of the History of Medicine*, 73 (1999), 429–446, at 434–5.

34. Wilkinson, *War*, 56.

35. Ibid. 54.

36. Thomas Robertson, 'Homeopathy and Post-War Reconstruction', *British Homeopathic Journal*, 32 (1942), 117.

37. Editorial, *British Homeopathic Journal*, 34 (1944), 157–210, at 157–8.

38. Correspondence, ibid. 186.

39. Dr Manasse, 'Homeopathy and General Practice', *British Homeopathic Journal*, 39 (1949), 186–7.

CHAPTER 3: 'THE CHINESE HAVE A GREAT DEAL OF WIT'

1. Francis Bacon, 'Masculine Birth of Time', trans. Benjamin Farrington, *The Philosophy of Francis Bacon* (Liverpool: Liverpool University Press, 1964), 61–133, at 62. The vast subjects of the Scientific Revolution and the Enlightenment have a correspondingly vast literature. So I'm going to list only my own favourite works on the subject; for a less idiosyncratic view, see the 'Further Reading' section. I love Charles Webster, *The Great Instauration* 2nd edn. (Oxford: Peter Lang, 2002); Steve Shapin and Simon Schaffer, *The Leviathan and the Air Pump* (Princeton: Princeton University Press, 1989); and Roy Porter's delicious *The Enlightenment* (Basingstoke: Palgrave, 2001).

2. Principal secondary sources for this chapter: Michael Adas, *Machines as the Measure of Men* (Ithaca: Cornell University Press, 1989); Robert A. Bickers (ed.), *Ritual and Diplomacy: The Macartney Mission to China, 1792–1794* (London: Wellsweep/British Association for Chinese Studies, 1993); Roberta Bivins, *Acupuncture, Expertise and Cross-Cultural Medicine* (Basingstoke: Palgrave, 2000); Nick Jewson, 'The Disappearance of the Sick Man from Medical Cosmology, 1770–1870', *Sociology*, 10 (1976), 225–44; Russell Maulitz, *Morbid Appearances: The Anatomy of Pathology in the Early Nineteenth Century* (Cambridge: Cambridge University Press, 1987); Stanley J. Reiser, *Medicine and the Reign of Technology* (Cambridge: Cambridge University Press: 1978); Kaufman, *Homeopathy* (see Chapter 2, n. 1); Nicholls, *Homeopathy*.

3. Sir John Floyer, *The Physician's Pulse-Watch*, 232 (see Introduction, n. 15).

4. J. B. DuHalde, *A Description of the Empire of China and Chinese-Tartary, . . . With Notes Geographical, Historical, and Critical; and Other Improvements, Particularly in the Maps, by the Translator*, ii (London: Edward Cave, 1741), 124.

5. Ibid. 235. My emphasis.

6. Abbé Jean-Baptiste Grosier, *A General Description of China . . . Together with the Latest Accounts which have Reached Europe, of the Government, Religion, Manners, Customs, Arts, and Sciences of the Chinese*, ii (London: G. G. J. and J. Robinson, 1787), 483–4.

7. Ibid.

8. L. V. J. Berlioz, *Mémoires sur les maladies chroniques, les évacuations sanguines et l'acupuncture* (Paris: Chez Croullebois, 1816), 150. All translations from this work are my own.

9. Ibid. 1.

10. 'Critical Analysis of English and Foreign Literature Relative to the Various Branches of Medical Science', *Medical and Physical Journal*, 48/286 (1822), 511–26, at 518.

11. R. James, *A Medicinal Dictionary*, i/1 (London: T. Osborne, 1743), no page numbers.

12. Scotus, 'Sciatica treated by Acupuncture with Dr. Alison's Opinion on the Mode of its Operation', *Lancet* (18 May 1827), 190–1.

13. Robley Dunglison, *New Remedies: Pharmaceutically and Therapeutically Considered; Fourth Edition with Extensive Modifications and Additions* (Philadelphia: Lea and Blanchard, 1843), 49.

14. William Buchan, *Observations Concerning the Prevention and Cure of Venereal Disease* (London: Chapman, 1796), p. iv.

15. Berlioz, *Mémoires*, 310–11.

16. Ibid. 296–7.

17. James Morss Churchill, *A Treatise on Acupuncturation* (London: Simpkin and Marshall, 1822), 5.

18. Ibid. 10.

19. Dunglison, *New Remedies*, 45–6.

20. T. W. Wansbrough, as quoted in James Morss Churchill, *Cases Illustrative of the Effects of Acupuncturation, in Rheumatism, Lumbago, Sciatica, Anomalous Muscular Diseases, and in Dropsy of the Cellular Tissue, etc.* (London: Callow and Wilson, 1828), 73–5.

21. C. Lindo, quoted ibid. 39–43.

22. Dunglison, *New Remedies*, 48.

23. Churchill, *Cases*, 46.

24. 'London Medical Society. March 18th, 1833. Mr. Kingdon, President. Rheumatism.—Elaterium. Acupuncture', *Lancet* (23 March 1833), 817–18, at 817.

25. Ibid.

26. See Steven Shapin and Simon Schaffer, *Leviathan and the Air-Pump* (see Chapter 3, n. 1) for more on the emergence of the culture of the witness, the audience, and the performance in science.

27. Churchill, *Treatise*, 23–4.

28. William Craig, 'Art. VII. Acupuncture in a Case of Cancer', *Edinburgh Medical Journal, Combining the Monthly Journal of Medicine and the Edinburgh Medical and Surgical Journal*, 14 (1869), 617–20, at 619.

29. T. Pridgin Teale, 'Clinical Essays, No. III. On the Relief of Pain and Muscular Disability by Acupuncture', *Lancet* (29 April 1871), 567–8, at 567.

30. Clarke Abel, *Narrative of a Journey in the Interior of China . . . in the Years 1816 and 1817; Containing an Account of the Most Interesting Transactions of Lord Amherst's Embassy to the Court of Pekin* (London: Longman, Hurst, Rees, Orme, and Brown, 1818), 107.

31. Ibid. 216.

32. 'Medicine in China' *Lancet*, 1(1838–9), 481–5.

33. The Opium Wars, also know as the Anglo-Chinese wars, were fought between 1839 and 1842, and 1856 and 1860, and as the name suggests, were sparked by China's decision to eradicate the highly profitable trade in opium dominated by the British. Opium, though known to be addictive and poisonous, was Britain's only successful export to China, and an effective ban would certainly have threatened Britain's balance in trade; however, Britain was anxious also to defend the right to free trade, and to eliminate the corrupt system under which Europeans were licensed to trade with China.

34. A Medical Practitioner, *Quacks and Quackery: A Remonstrance against the Sanction given by the Government, the Press, and the Public, to the System of Imposture and Fraud Practised on the Ignorant and Credulous in the Quackeries of the Day* (London: Simpkin, Marshall and Co., 1844), 30–1.

35. John Wilson, *Medical Notes on China* (London: John Churchill, 1846) 248.

CHAPTER 4: 'WITH OUR WESTERN BRETHREN, THE CASE SEEMS TO BE QUITE DIFFERENT'

1. Principal secondary sources for this chapter: David Arnold, *Colonizing the Body: State Medicine and Epidemic Diseases in Nineteenth Century India* (Berkeley and Los Angeles: University of California Press, 1993); M. N. Pearson, 'First Contacts between Indian and European Medical Systems: Goa in the Sixteenth Century', in David Arnold (ed.), *Warm Climates and Western Medicine* (Amsterdam: Rodopi, 1996), 20–41; Waltraud Ernst (ed.), *Plural Medicine, Tradition and Modernity, 1800–2000* (London: Routledge, 2002); Winter, *Mesmerized*, 187–212 (see Chapter 2, n. 1); Michael Worboys, *Spreading Germs: Disease Theories and Medical Practice in Britain, 1865–1900* (Cambridge: Cambridge University Press, 2000).

2. *Indian Medical Gazette* (1887), quoted in Arnold, *Colonizing the Body*, 135.

3. John Fryer, *A New Account of India and Persia*, i (London: Hakluyt Society, 1909–15), 180.

4. *Breve Relação dans escrituras dos gentios da India Oriental a dos sues costumes* (1812), quoted in Pearson, 'First Contacts', 26–7.

5. William Jones, 'A Discourse on the Institution of a Society for Inquiring into the History, Civil and Natural, the Antiquities, Arts, Sciences, and Literature, of Asia', *Asiatick Researches; Or, Transactions of the Society Instituted in Bengal, for Inquiring into the History and Antiquities, the Arts, Sciences, and Literature, of Asia*, 1, 5th edn. (1806), pp. ix–xvi, at pp. xiii–xiv.

6. William Jones, 'The Second Anniversary Discourse, delivered 24th February, 1785', *Asiatick Researches* 403–414, at 408–9.

7. Francis Buchanan, 'Journal of Progress and Observations during the Continuance of the Deputation from Bengal to Ava in 1795 in the Dominions of the Barma [*sic*] Monarch', 2 vols. British Library MS Eur. C. 12, 13. Dc. 1.74: 248.

8. R. H. Irvine, 'On the Materia Medica of Amjer; in a Letter to the Secretary to the Committee of Inquiry upon the Vegetable, Animal and Mineral Productions of Medicinal Qualities procurable in India and the Surrounding Countries', *Quarterly Journal of the Calcutta Medical and Physical Society*, 6 (1 Apr., 1838), 191–223, at 191.

9. In India, variolation took the form of the introduction into the nose or onto abraded skin of aged, powdered matter gathered from the pox of a mild case of smallpox. The individual, usually a child, being inoculated was specially prepared for the procedure both physically and spiritually, and the variolation was performed at a particularly auspicious time.

10. Both cited in Arnold, *Colonizing the Body*, 136.

11. Conférence Sanitaire Internationale (1866), cited ibid. 187.

12. W. W. Hunter, *Orissa* (1872), cited ibid. 189.

13. F. S. Roberts (1892), cited ibid. 196.

14. *Kalapataru* (1897) and *Vartahar* (1898), both cited ibid. 214-15.

15. This use of the term, originally used to describe European scholars of the Middle East and then of Asia generally in the late eighteenth and early nineteenth century, derives from Edward Said, *Orientalism: Western Conceptions of the Orient* (New York: Pantheon Books, 1978).

16. James Esdaile, *Mesmerism in India, and its Practical Application in Surgery and Medicine* (London: Longman, Brown, Green and Longmans, 1846), 14-15.

17. Quoted in Winter, *Mesmerized*, 199.

18. Esdaile, *Mesmerism in India*, 14-15.

19. James Esdaile, *The Introduction of Mesmerism (with the Sanction of the Government) into the Public Hospitals of India* (London: W. Kent and Co., 1856), 14.

20. 'Letter from the Marquis of Dalhousie to the Poor Law Guardians of Exeter', in Esdaile, *Mesmerism in India*, 4.

21. F. C. Skipwith, *Calcutta Review* (1852), quoted in David Arnold and Sumit Sarkar, 'In Search of Rational Remedies: Homeopathy in Nineteenth Century Bengal', in Ernst (ed.), *Plural Medicine*, 40-57, at 42.

22. 'Mr. Kingdon on Homeopathy', *Journal of the Calcutta Medical and Physical Society* 1(1 July 1837), 405.

23. Ibid.

24. G. Srinivasamurti, 'Appendix I. A Memorandum on the science and the art of Indian Medicine', *Report of the Committee on the Indigenous Systems of Medicine, Madras* (Madras: Government of Madras, 1923), 62.

25. See Gary Hausman, 'Making Medicine Indigenous: Homeopathy in South India', *Social History of Medicine*, 15/2 (2002), 303-22; Arnold and Sarkar, 'In Search of Rational Remedies', 40-57.

26. Quoted in Arnold and Sarkar, 'In Search of Rational Remedies', 46.

27. Quoted ibid. 44-5.

28. Quoted in *Report of the Committee on the Indigenous Systems of Medicine, Madras*, 8.

29. See Richard Evans, *Death in Hamburg: Society and Politics in the Cholera Years, 1830-1910* (Oxford: Clarendon Press, 1987): 497-8.

30. Quoted in Nancy Tomes, *Gospel of Germs: Men, Women and the Microbe in American Life* (Cambridge, Mass.: Harvard Univeristy Press, 1998), 26.

31. *Lancet* (2 Feb. 1895), 297.
32. Ibid.
33. Worboys, *Spreading Germs*, ch. 7, Conclusion.
34. Government Order No. 1351, 21 Feb. 1921.
35. See Claudia Leibeskind, 'Arguing Science: Unani tibb, Hakims, and Biomedicine in India, 1900–1950' in Ernst (ed.), *Plural Medicine*, 58–75.
36. Muhammad Usman, *Report of the Committee on the Indigenous Systems of Medicine, Madras*, 1.
37. Srinivasamurti, 'Appendix I', 40.
38. Usman, *Report*, 10.
39. Ibid. 11.
40. Srinivasamurti, 'Appendix I'.
41. Ibid. 30–2.
42. Ibid. 41.
43. For this and the quotes which follow, see ibid. 42–3.

CONCLUSION: PRAGMATISM, PLURALISM, AND THE (IM)PATIENT-CONSUMER

1. Principal secondary sources for this chapter include: Hans Baer, *Biomedicine and Alternative Healing Systems in America: Issues of Class, Race, Ethnicity, and Gender* (Madison: University of Wisconsin Press, 2001); Roberta Bivins, 'Acupuncture and Innovation: "New Age" Medicine in the NHS', in Jennifer Stanton (ed.), *Innovations in Health and Medicine* (London: Routledge, 2002), 84–105; Phil Fontanarosa (ed.), *Alternative Medicine: An Objective Assessment* (Chicago: American Medical Association, 2000); Sam King, *Tiger Balm King: The Life and Times of Aw Boon Har* (Singapore: Times Books International, 1992); Ursula Sharma, *Complementary Medicine Today: Patients and Practitioners*, rev. edn. (London: Routledge, 1995); Charles Vincent and Adrian Furnham, *Complementary Medicine: A Research Perspective* (Chichester, John Wiley and Sons, 1997).
2. www.tigerbalm.com/02_whatis.htm and www.hawpar.com/heritage.htm respectively; both accessed 26 Feb. 2005.
3. A process which continues with unabated avidity today, as evidenced by the popularity of guided tours of major Chinatowns like those in London, New York, and San Francisco, and by television programmes too numerous to list separately.
4. Diphtheria is a bacterial disease of childhood; under epidemic conditions it killed up to half of all infected children, either through suffocation by the leathery membrane it produces on the pharyngeal

tissues, or by its paralysing toxin. The infective organism was identified in 1883, anti-diphtheria toxin was first produced in 1890, and now children across the developed world are routinely immunized. Even with antibiotics, anti-toxin, and modern airway maintenance, 5 per cent of children infected by a virulent strain today still die of the disease. In 1872 diphtheria killed 600 people in Victoria. See Rey Tiquia, 'Learning from the Chinese' Lateline TV programme transcript, accessed on 24 Jan. 2006 at http://www.abc.net.au/lateline/content/2003/hc12.htm; and Rey Tiquia, 'Regulating and Evaluating TCM: Learning from the Diphtheria Controversy of the 1870s', unpublished paper, read at the SSHM Annual Conference 'Plural Medicine: Orthodox and Heterodox Medicine in Western and Colonial Countries, during the 19th and 20th centuries,', 15 Sept. 1998. This material, including all quotations, has been taken from these two sources.

5. Burn J. Malcolm, 'Letter, June 25th, 1870', *Australian Medical Journal*, (1870) 221–2, quoted in Tiquia, 'Plural Medicine', 7–8.

6. Parliament of Victoria Debate, 13 Aug. 1874, p. 904, quoted ibid. 8–9.

7. This and subsequent quotations from Stewart Culin, 'The Practice of Medicine by the Chinese in America' (Philadelphia), Pamphlet reprn. from the *Medical and Surgical Reporter* (19 Mar. 1887), 1–3. Culin also described one of the crucial problems in assessing the medical expertise of any culture based on the practices of immigrants: 'The doctors, called *i shang*, of whom there are now four in Philadelphia, are usually from the Sam Yap, or "Three Districts" immediately adjacent to Canton city. They are much better educated than the mass of the people. None of any repute at home come to America, but it is said there are several very skilful ones in San Francisco and some of the western cities, who have a large practice among Americans. Those of New York and Philadelphia rank very low in their profession, in the estimation of their countrymen.'

8. Unfortunately, there is insufficient space in this volume to explore these topics in depth. To explore these questions, see e.g. Amy Fairchild, *Science at the Borders: Immigrant Medical Inspection and the Shaping of the Modern Industrial Labor Force* (Baltimore: Johns Hopkins University Press, 2003); Colin Holms, *John Bull's Island: Immigration and British Society, 1871–1971* (London: Macmillan, 1988); Lara Marks and Michael Worboys (eds.), *Migrants, Minorities and Health* (London: Routledge, 1997); Nayan Shah, *Contagious Divides: Epidemics and Race in San Francisco's Chinatown* (Berkeley and Los Angeles, University of California Press,

2001); Alexandra Minna Stern, *Eugenic Nation: Faults and Frontiers of Better Breeding in Modern America* (Berkeley and Los Angeles: University of California Press, 2005).

9. David Eisenberg, Roger Davis, Susan Ettner, Scott Appel, Sonya Wilkey, Maria Van Rompay, Ronald Kessler, 'Trends in Alternative Medicine Use in the United States, 1990–1997', in Fontanarosa (ed.), *Alternative Medicine*, 4–15.

10. Francis Peabody, 'The Care of the Patient' *JAMA* 88 (1927), 877–82. In 1997, these sentiments still resounded with segments of the medical community; in a lecture delivered to students at Williams College in the United States, John Balint (a prominent medical scientist and ethicist) argued: 'In our love affair with Science we have forgotten that the endpoint of medicine is to make people happy, to be co-factors in helping to improve lives.' John Balint, quoted in David Elpern, 'Beyond Complementary and Alternative Medicine', in Fontanarosa (ed.), *Alternative Medicine,* 566–70, at 569.

11. Christopher Driver, 'The Tiger Balm Community', *Manchester Guardian*, 2 Jan. 1962.

12. e.g. Margaret Naeser, *Outline Guide to Chinese Herbal Patent Medicine in Pill Form* (Boston: Boston Chinese Medicine, 1990).

13. Eisenberg et al., 'Trends in Alternative Medicine Use', 4–15.

14. Elpern, 'Beyond Complementary and Allopathic Medicine', 569.

15. House of Lords Select Committee on Science and Technology, *Complementary and Alternative Medicine* (London: HMSO, 2000) 15.

16. Gry Sagli, 'Chinese Medical Concepts in Biomedical Culture: The Case of Acupuncture in Norway', in Robert Jütte, Motzi Eklöf, and Marie C. Nelson (eds.), *Historical Aspects of Unconventional Medicine: Approaches, Concepts, Case Studies* (Sheffield: European Association for the History of Medicine and Health Publications, 2001), 211–26. Sagli's survey, performed in 1995 by postal questionnaire of 435 people, including all 274 listed in yellow pages under acupuncture for entire country elicited an 80 per cent response rate. The final data represent information gathered from the questionnaires of 298 active practitioners. These practitioners were divided into four groups: medical doctors (57), physiotherapists (138), others trained as 'authorised health personnel' (37), and practitioners with no training as 'authorised health personnel' (66).

17. Ibid. 216.

18. Ibid. 217.

19. Ibid. 218.

20. For a detailed description of the dissemination of acupuncture practice in nineteenth-century Britain, see Bivins, *Acupuncture, Expertise and Cross-Cultural Medicine*, esp. chs. 3 and 4.

21. National Medical Advisory Committee (NMAC), *Complementary Medicine and the National Health Service: An Examination of Acupuncture, Homeopathy, Chiropractic and Osteopathy* (Edinburgh: HMSO, 1997) 9.

22. Ibid. 16.

23. Thomas Reardon, 'Preface', in Fontanarosa (ed.), *Alternative Medicine*, p. v.

24. Wayne Jonas, 'Alternative Medicine—Learning from the Past, Examining the Present, Advancing to the Future', *JAMA* 280 (1998), 1616–18.

25. Sharma, *Complementary Medicine Today*, 28–9; A. Minocha, 'Medical Pluralism and Health Services', *Social Sciences and Medicine*, 14B (1980), 217–23.

26. Quotations and images in this section drawn from Pandit D. Gopalacharlu, *Descriptive Price List of Patent and Other Sastric Medicines, Scientifically Prepared at the Madras Ayurvedic Laboratory . . . With a Historical Sketch of Ayurveda*, 10th edn. (Madras: Madras Ayurvedic Laboratory, 1909).

27. Quoted ibid. 25.

28. Quoted ibid. 24–5.

29. Sarat Chandra Ghose, 'Ayurvedic Medicine', *Medical Times* (Jan. 1917), 28–32.

30. This and succeeding quotations all from 'Systems of Medicine', *Lancet* (23 May 1964), 1144–6.

31. Sohan Singh Hayreh, 'Letters', *Lancet* (6 June 1964), 1275–6.

32. Janet McKee, 'Holistic Health and the Critique of Western Medicine', *Social Science and Medicine*, 26/8 (1988), 775–84, at 775.

INDEX

The Index includes the Introduction, Chapters 1–4 and the Conclusion, but not the Further Reading or Notes. Filing order is word-by-word.